34124-01002369-2

Living with Bipolar Disorder

Dr Neel Burton qualified in medicine from King's College, London, and is a Member of the Royal College of Psychiatrists. He is the principal author of three other books, including a textbook of psychiatry and a self-help book on schizophrenia, *Living with Schizophrenia* (Sheldon Press, 2007), which recently won a national award for 'best self-help book'. His recent book, *The Meaning of Madness*, published by Acheron Press, explores what mental disorders can teach us about human nature and the human condition.

D1471570

Overcoming Common Problems Series

Selected titles

A full list of titles is available from Sheldon Press,
36 Causton Street, London SW1P 4ST and on our website at
www.sheldonpress.co.uk

The Assertiveness Handbook
Mary Hartley

Assertiveness: Step by step
Dr Windy Dryden and Daniel Constantinou

Body Language: What you need to know
David Cohen

Breaking Free
Carolyn Ainscough and Kay Toon

Calm Down
Paul Hauck

The Candida Diet Book
Karen Brody

Cataract: What you need to know
Mark Watts

The Chronic Fatigue Healing Diet
Christine Craggs-Hinton

The Chronic Pain Diet Book
Neville Shone

Cider Vinegar
Margaret Hills

The Complete Carer's Guide
Bridget McCall

The Confidence Book
Gordon Lamont

Confidence Works
Gladeana McMahon

Coping Successfully with Pain
Neville Shone

Coping Successfully with Panic Attacks
Shirley Trickett

Coping Successfully with Period Problems
Mary-Claire Mason

Coping Successfully with Psoriasis
Christine Craggs-Hinton

Coping Successfully with Ulcerative Colitis
Peter Cartwright

Coping Successfully with Varicose Veins
Christine Craggs-Hinton

Coping Successfully with Your Hiatus Hernia
Dr Tom Smith

Coping Successfully with Your Irritable Bowel
Rosemary Nicol

Coping with Age-related Memory Loss
Dr Tom Smith

Coping with Alopecia
Dr Nigel Hunt and Dr Sue McHale

Coping with Birth Trauma and Postnatal Depression
Lucy Jolin

Coping with Bowel Cancer
Dr Tom Smith

Coping with Brain Injury
Maggie Rich

Coping with Candida
Shirley Trickett

Coping with Chemotherapy
Dr Terry Priestman

Coping with Childhood Allergies
Jill Eckersley

Coping with Childhood Asthma
Jill Eckersley

Coping with Chronic Fatigue
Trudie Chalder

Coping with Coeliac Disease
Karen Brody

Coping with Compulsive Eating
Ruth Searle

Coping with Diabetes in Childhood and Adolescence
Dr Philippa Kaye

Coping with Diverticulitis
Peter Cartwright

Coping with Down's Syndrome
Fiona Marshall

Coping with Dyspraxia
Jill Eckersley

Overcoming Common Problems Series

Overcoming Common Problems Series

Living with Crohn's Disease
Dr Joan Gomez

Living with Eczema
Jill Eckersley

Living with Fibromyalgia
Christine Craggs-Hinton

Living with Food Intolerance
Alex Gazzola

Living with Grief
Dr Tony Lake

Living with Heart Failure
Susan Elliot-Wright

Living with Loss and Grief
Julia Tugendhat

Living with Lupus
Philippa Pigache

Living with Osteoarthritis
Dr Patricia Gilbert

Living with Osteoporosis
Dr Joan Gomez

Living with Rheumatoid Arthritis
Philippa Pigache

Living with Schizophrenia
Dr Neel Burton and Dr Phil Davison

Living with a Seriously Ill Child
Dr Jan Aldridge

Living with Sjögren's Syndrome
Sue Dyson

Losing a Baby
Sarah Ewing

Losing a Child
Linda Hurcombe

The Multiple Sclerosis Diet Book
Tessa Buckley

Osteoporosis: Prevent and treat
Dr Tom Smith

Overcoming Agoraphobia
Melissa Murphy

Overcoming Anorexia
Professor J. Hubert Lacey, Christine Craggs-Hinton and Kate Robinson

Overcoming Anxiety
Dr Windy Dryden

Overcoming Back Pain
Dr Tom Smith

Overcoming Depression
Dr Windy Dryden and Sarah Opie

Overcoming Emotional Abuse
Susan Elliot-Wright

Overcoming Hurt
Dr Windy Dryden

Overcoming Insomnia
Susan Elliot-Wright

Overcoming Jealousy
Dr Windy Dryden

Overcoming Procrastination
Dr Windy Dryden

Overcoming Shyness and Social Anxiety
Ruth Searle

Overcoming Tiredness and Exhaustion
Fiona Marshall

The PMS Handbook
Theresa Cheung

Reducing Your Risk of Cancer
Dr Terry Priestman

Safe Dieting for Teens
Linda Ojeda

The Self-Esteem Journal
Alison Waines

Simplify Your Life
Naomi Saunders

Stammering: Advice for all ages
Renée Byrne and Louise Wright

Stress-related Illness
Dr Tim Cantopher

Ten Steps to Positive Living
Dr Windy Dryden

Think Your Way to Happiness
Dr Windy Dryden and Jack Gordon

The Thinking Person's Guide to Happiness
Ruth Searle

Tranquillizers and Antidepressants: When to start them, how to stop
Professor Malcolm Lader

The Traveller's Good Health Guide
Dr Ted Lankester

Treating Arthritis Diet Book
Margaret Hills

Treating Arthritis: The drug-free way
Margaret Hills

Treating Arthritis: More drug-free ways
Margaret Hills

Understanding Obsessions and Compulsions
Dr Frank Tallis

When Someone You Love Has Depression
Barbara Baker

Overcoming Common Problems

Living with Bipolar Disorder

DR NEEL BURTON

WESTERN ISLES LIBRARIES	
34134010023692	
Bertrams	03/12/2014
616.895	£8.99

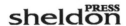

First published in Great Britain in 2009

Sheldon Press
36 Causton Street
London SW1P 4ST

Copyright © Neel Burton 2009

All rights reserved. No part of this book may be reproduced or
transmitted in any form or by any means, electronic or mechanical,
including photocopying, recording, or by any information storage and
retrieval system, without permission in writing from the publisher.

The author and publisher have made every effort to ensure that the
external website and email addresses included in this book are correct and
up to date at the time of going to press. The author and publisher are not
responsible for the content, quality or continuing accessibility of the sites.

The extract from the Authorized Version of the Bible (The King James
Bible), the rights in which are vested in the Crown, is reproduced by
permission of the Crown's Patentee, Cambridge University Press.

British Library Cataloguing-in-Publication Data
A catalogue record for this book is available from the British Library

ISBN 978–1–84709–054–6

1 3 5 7 9 10 8 6 4 2

Typeset by Fakenham Photosetting Ltd, Fakenham, Norfolk
Printed in Great Britain by Ashford Colour Press

Produced on paper from sustainable forests

*This book is dedicated to bipolar sufferers and to their carers,
on whom they and we depend*

Contents

Note: This is not a medical book and is not intended to replace advice from your doctor. Do consult with your doctor if you are experiencing symptoms with which you feel you need help.

True, we love life, not because we are used to living, but because we are used to loving. There is always some madness in love, but there is also always some reason in madness.

Friedrich Nietzsche, *Thus Spake Zarathustra*

Foreword

Coping effectively with bipolar disorder involves being honest and realistic, making sensible lifestyle changes, and working in partnership with health-care professionals. Knowledge of the illness and of its treatments is the foundation stone for all of these coping strategies.

Dr Neel Burton's book, *Living with Bipolar Disorder*, provides an excellent overview of the important topics. It explains what is currently known about the illness, its causes and triggers, the treatments available, and the lifestyle changes that can make a real difference. It is invaluable reading for anyone who has been diagnosed with bipolar disorder, for his or her family and friends, and for all those who want to find out more about the illness.

I have no doubt whatsoever that this book will be of tremendous help to all those who are living with bipolar disorder.

Nick Craddock
Professor of Psychiatry, Cardiff University
Scientific Adviser to MDF the Bipolar Organization
Principal Researcher, Bipolar Disorder Research Network

Introduction

Bipolar disorder is a disorder of mood. Broadly speaking, mood disorders can be divided into unipolar disorders and bipolar disorders. To meet the criteria for having a bipolar disorder, a person must have had one or more episodes of abnormally elevated mood (mania or hypomania). If a person has only ever had episodes of abnormally depressed mood, then he or she has a unipolar disorder unless and until he or she develops an episode of abnormally elevated mood. The unipolar–bipolar distinction is an important one to make, because the course and treatment of bipolar disorders differ significantly from those of unipolar disorders.

Episodes of mania are characterized by elevated or irritable mood and often also by decreased need for sleep, inflated self-esteem or grandiosity, agitation, racing thoughts, increased talkativeness, distractibility, and impulsive and risk-taking behaviour. In severe cases, there may also be psychotic symptoms, such as delusions and hallucinations, which involve a profound distortion of reality.

People who have had one or more manic episodes typically also experience episodes of abnormally depressed mood ('depression'), and sometimes also mixed episodes characterized by features of both mania *and* depression. In some cases, episodes of depression in bipolar disorder can be severe and involve both suicidal thoughts and psychotic symptoms. Thus psychotic symptoms can be a feature of both manic and depressive episodes, as well as of other psychotic illnesses such as schizophrenia and schizoaffective disorder. In bipolar disorder, manic and depressive episodes may last from several days to several months, and are usually separated by periods of normal mood.

The length of these periods of normal mood can vary a lot from one person to another and from one period to the next.

To a large extent, the goal of treatment is to extend periods of normal mood for as long as possible by stabilizing mood and preventing further episodes of mood disorder. In some cases, particularly if a person does all the right things, relapses may not recur for several years, if at all. I hope that this book will give you and your relatives the expertise and confidence to do all of these right things, and thereby to take control over an illness that can be as frightening as it is damaging.

Dr Neel Burton

1

What's in a name?
(Bipolar disorder through history)

How was bipolar disorder perceived in ancient times?

In antiquity, people used the term 'madness' to refer indiscriminately to all forms of psychosis, that is, the psychosis of schizophrenia and the 'affective psychoses' of mania and depression. In those days, they did not think of 'madness' in terms of mental illness, but in terms of divine punishment or demonic possession. Evidence for this comes from the Old Testament, for example, from the First Book of Samuel, which relates how King Saul became 'mad' after neglecting his religious duties and angering God. The fact that David used to play on his harp to make Saul better suggests that, even in antiquity, people believed that psychotic illnesses could be successfully treated.

> But the spirit of the LORD departed from Saul, and an evil spirit from the LORD troubled him.

> And it came to pass, when the evil spirit from God was upon Saul, that David took an harp, and played with his hand: so Saul was refreshed, and was well, and the evil spirit departed from him.
>
> 1 Samuel 16.14, 16.23

When did people first start thinking of bipolar disorder as an illness?

In Greek mythology and the Homerian epics, madness is similarly thought of as a punishment from God, or the gods. Thus Hera punishes Hercules by 'sending madness upon him', and Agamemnon confides to Achilles that 'Zeus robbed me of my

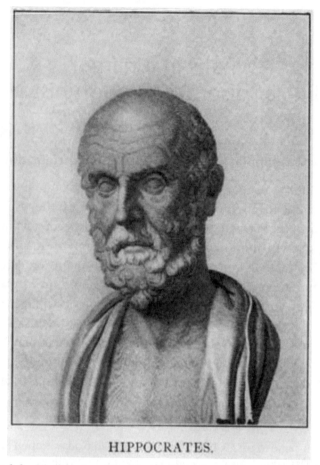

HIPPOCRATES.

Figure 1.1 Hippocrates. Courtesy of the National Library of Medicine.

wits'. It is in actual fact not until the time of the Greek physician Hippocrates (460–377 BC) that mental illness first became an object of scientific speculation. Hippocrates (see Figure 1.1) thought that mental illness resulted from an imbalance of four bodily humours and that it could be cured by rebalancing these humours with such treatments as special diets, purgatives and blood-lettings. To modern readers Hippocrates' ideas may seem far-fetched, perhaps even on the dangerous side of eccentric, but in the fourth century BC they represented a significant advance on the idea of mental illness as a punishment from God. The Greek philosopher Aristotle (384–322 BC) and later the Roman physician Galen (129–216 AD) expanded on Hippocrates' humoural theories, and both men played an important role in establishing them as Europe's dominant medical model.

> Only from the brain springs our pleasures, our feelings of happiness, laughter and jokes, our pain, our sorrows and tears ... This same organ makes us mad or confused, inspires us with fear and anxiety...

It is of particular interest to note that not all people in Ancient Greece invariably thought of 'madness' as a curse or an illness. In Plato's *Phaedrus*, the Greek philosopher Socrates (470–399 BC) has this to say:

> Madness, provided it comes as the gift of heaven, is the channel by which we receive the greatest blessings ... the men of old who gave things their names saw no disgrace or reproach in madness; otherwise they would not have connected it with the name of the noblest of arts, the art of discerning the future, and called it the manic art. ... So, according to the evidence provided by our ancestors, madness is a nobler thing than sober sense ... madness comes from God, whereas sober sense is merely human.

In Ancient Rome, the physician Asclepiades and the statesman and philosopher Cicero (106–43 BC) rejected Hippocrates' humoural theories, asserting, for example, that melancholy resulted not from an excess of black bile but from emotions such as rage, fear, and grief. Unfortunately, in the first century AD the influence of Asclepiades and Cicero started to decline, and the Roman physician Celsus reinstated the idea of madness as a punishment from the gods – an idea to be later reinforced by the rise of Christianity and the collapse of the Roman Empire. In the Middle Ages religion became central to cure and, alongside the mediaeval asylums such as the Bethlehem in London, some monasteries transformed themselves into centres for the treatment of mental illness. This is not to say that the humoural theories of Hippocrates had been forgotten. Instead, they had been incorporated into the prevailing Christian beliefs, and the purgatives and blood-lettings continued alongside the prayers and confession.

How did these beliefs change?

The burning of the so-called heretics – often people suffering from psychotic illnesses such as schizophrenia and bipolar disorder – began in the early Renaissance and reached its peak in the fourteenth and fifteenth centuries. *De praestigiis daemonum et incantationibus ac venificiis* (On the deception of demons and on spells and poisons), which was first published in 1563, argued that the madness of 'heretics' resulted not from divine punishment or demonic possession, but from natural causes. The

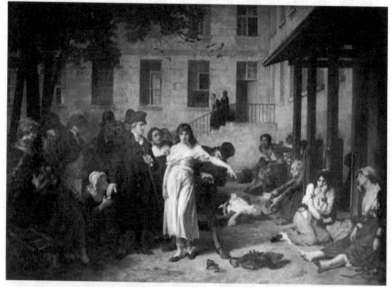

Figure 1.2 In this 1876 painting by Tony Robert-Fleury, Pinel is seen freeing people with mental illness from the confinements of the old asylums. (Charcot Library, Salpêtrière Hospital Medical School, Paris.)

Church banned the book and accused its author, Johann Weyer, of being a sorcerer. From the fifteenth century, scientific break-throughs such as those of the astronomer Galileo (1564–1642) and the anatomist Vesalius (1514–1584) began challenging the authority of the Church, and the centre of attention and study gradually shifted from God to man, and from the heavens to the earth. Unfortunately this did not translate into better treatments and so Hippocrates' humoural theories persisted up to and into the eighteenth century. Empirical thinkers such as John Locke (1632–1704) in England and Denis Diderot (1713–1784) in France challenged this status quo by arguing that reason and emotions are caused by sensations. Also in France, the physician Philippe Pinel (1745–1826) began to regard mental illness as the result of exposure to psychological and social stresses. A landmark in the history of psychiatry, Pinel's *Medico-Philosophical Treatise on Mental Alienation or Mania*, called for a more humane approach to the treatment of mental illness. This so-called 'moral treat-ment' included respect for the person, a trusting and confiding doctor–patient relationship, decreased stimuli, routine activity, and the abandonment of old-fashioned Hippocratic treatments (see Figure 1.2). At about the same time as Pinel in France, the Tukes (father and son) in England founded the York Retreat, the first institution 'for the humane care of the insane' in the British Isles.

Who 'discovered' bipolar disorder?

The terms used for the bipolar extremes – 'melancholy' (depres-sion) and 'mania' – both have their origins in Ancient Greek. 'Melancholy' derives from *melas*, 'black', and *chole*, 'bile', because Hippocrates thought that depression resulted from an excess of black bile. 'Mania' is related to *menos*, 'spirit, force, passion', *mainesthai*, 'to rage, to go mad', and *mantis*, 'seer', and ultimately derives from the Indo-European root *men-*, 'mind'.

('Depression', the clinical term for melancholy, is much more recent and derives from the Latin *deprimere*, 'to press down' or 'to sink down'.)

The idea of a relationship between melancholy and mania can be traced back to the Ancient Greeks, and particularly to Aretaeus of Cappadocia, who was a physician and philosopher in the time of Nero, or Vespasian, who also lived in the first century AD. Aretaeus described a group of patients that would 'laugh, play, dance night and day, and sometimes go openly to the market crowned, as if victors in some contest of skill', only to be 'torpid, dull, and sorrowful' at other times. Aretaeus suggested that both patterns of behaviour resulted from one and the same illness, but this idea did not gain currency until the modern era.

Instead, the modern psychiatric concept of manic–depressive illness has its origins in the nineteenth century. In 1854, Jules Baillarger (1809–1890) and Jean-Pierre Falret (1794–1870) inde-pendently presented descriptions of manic–depressive illness to the *Académie de Médicine* in Paris. Baillarger called the illness *folie à double forme* (dual-form insanity) and Falret called it *folie circu-laire* (circular insanity). Falret observed that the illness clustered in families, and correctly postulated that it had a strong genetic basis. In the early 1900s the eminent German psychiatrist Emil Kraepelin (1856–1926) studied the natural course of untreated bipolar patients and found the illness to be punctuated by rela-tively symptom-free intervals. He distinguished the illness from schizophrenia, and coined the term 'manic–depressive psychosis' to describe it. Kraepelin emphasized that, in contrast to schizo-phrenia, manic–depressive illness had a periodic or episodic course and a more benign outcome. However, Kraepelin did not distin-guish between people with both manic and depressive episodes, and those with unipolar depressive episodes with psychotic symp-toms. This distinction dates back only to the 1960s; it is largely responsible for the modern emphasis on bipolarity – and hence on mania, or mood elevation – as the defining feature of the illness.

The terms 'manic–depressive illness' and 'bipolar disorder' are comparatively recent, and date from the 1950s and 1980s, respectively. The term 'bipolar disorder' (or 'bipolar affective disorder') is thought to be less stigmatizing than the older 'manic–depressive illness', and so 'bipolar disorder' has largely superseded 'manic–depressive illness'. That having been said, some psychiatrists and bipolar sufferers still prefer 'manic–depressive illness' because they feel that it better describes the nature of the illness.

Were there any effective treatments for bipolar disorder at that time?

Even though the modern psychiatric concept of bipolar disorder has its origins in the nineteenth century, the first effective treatments for the illness did not appear until the second half of the twentieth century. Febrile illnesses such as malaria had been observed to temper psychotic symptoms, and in the early twentieth century fever therapy became a popular form of treatment for psychotic illnesses. Psychiatrists tried to induce fevers in their patients, sometimes even by means of injections of sulphur or oil. Other popular but unsatisfactory treatments included sleep therapy, electroconvulsive therapy, and prefrontal leukotomy – the destruction of the part of the brain that processes emotions. Sadly, many such 'treatments' were aimed more at controlling disturbed behaviour than at curing illness or alleviating suffering. Then in 1948, the Australian psychiatrist and researcher John Cade serendipitously discovered the calming properties of lithium, and this naturally occurring substance became the first effective treatment for bipolar disorder.

Lithium opened up an era of hope and promise for bipolar sufferers and their carers. Since the advent of lithium and other mood stabilizers, old-fashioned treatments have all but disappeared. The one treatment that has survived in a greatly modified form is electroconvulsive therapy, because it has been demonstrated to be safe and effective in the treatment of mental illnesses involving mood symptoms that are both severe and unresponsive to medication. However, compared with lithium and other mood stabilizers, modern electroconvulsive therapy is only rarely used.

Our ever-increasing understanding of bipolar disorder has opened up multiple avenues for the treatment of the illness, and there are now a broad range of pharmacological, psychological, and social treatments that have been scientifically proven to be effective. Today, bipolar sufferers stand a better chance than at any other time in history of leading a healthy and productive life. And thanks to the fast pace of ongoing medical research, a good outcome is increasingly likely.

2

Who is affected by bipolar disorder, and why?

Many people with bipolar disorder and their families do not talk openly about the condition, for fear of being misunderstood or stigmatized. This deplorable state of affairs can lead to the impression that bipolar disorder is an uncommon, even a rare, illness.

In fact, bipolar disorder is so common that most people will know of someone with the illness. The chance of any given person developing bipolar disorder in his or her lifetime is about 1 per cent (or one in 100).

Why is such a terrible illness so common?

Genes for potentially debilitating illnesses usually become less common over time: the fact that this hasn't happened for bipolar disorder suggests that the genes responsible are being selected despite their potentially debilitating effects on a significant proportion of the population. The reason for this could be that the genes confer important adaptive advantages to our species, such as the abilities for language and creativity. Such abilities not only set us clearly apart from other animals, but also make us extremely adept at the game of survival.

A significant number of highly creative people have suffered from bipolar disorder, including Ernest Hemingway, John Keats, Sylvia Plath, Robert Schumann, and Virginia Woolf. In *Touched with Fire: Manic Depressive Illness and the Artistic Temperament*, Professor Kay Redfield Jamison – who herself suffers from the illness – estimates that bipolar disorder is between 10 and 40 times more common among artists than among the general public. It must be stressed that such artists tend to be at their most creative not during relapses of the illness, but during periods of remission when symptoms are either mild or absent.

> I am come of a race noted for vigor of fancy and ardour of passion. Men have called me mad; but the question is not yet settled, whether madness is or is not the loftiest intelligence – whether much that is glorious – whether all that is profound – does not spring from disease of thought – from moods of mind exalted at the expense of the general intellect. They who dream by day are cognizant of many things which escape those who dream only by night. In their grey visions they obtain glimpses of eternity … They penetrate, however rudderless or compassless, into the vast ocean of the 'light ineffable'.
>
> Edgar Allen Poe, *Eleonora*

It is not just people with bipolar disorder who are more creative than average, but also their relatives who share some of their genes. People who are more creative than average tend to be more successful than average, and this no doubt explains the finding that bipolar disorder is particularly common in people from higher socio-economic groups.

At what age does bipolar disorder first develop?

Bipolar disorder can present at any age, but it is rare in childhood and early adolescence. Most cases are diagnosed in late adolescence or early adulthood, with a median age of onset of about 21 years and a mean age of onset of about 30 years. If symptoms indicative of bipolar disorder occur for the first time in middle or old age, it is particularly important for the psychiatrist to exclude other conditions that can present like bipolar disorder (see Table 4.1, page 32). This is not only because such conditions are more common in older people, but also because it is relatively uncommon for bipolar disorder to develop so late.

In some cases, a person may have one or several depressive episodes before eventually developing a manic episode several years later and 'uncovering' a diagnosis of bipolar disorder. The initial diagnosis of depressive disorder or recurrent depressive disorder is then revised to one of bipolar disorder, even though the person in question had bipolar disorder all along. This is because it is impossible to diagnose bipolar disorder unless there has been evidence of a manic or hypomanic episode (see pp. 23–5). That having been said, a diagnosis of bipolar disorder should be suspected in anyone with a depressive disorder and a strong family history of bipolar disorder.

Are both sexes equally affected?

Unlike many other mental illnesses such as depression and anxiety disorders, which tend to be significantly more common in women, bipolar disorder affects men and women in more or less equal numbers. However, the first onset of mania tends to be later in women, who are also more likely to have more depressive episodes, mixed episodes characterized by concurrent symptoms of both mania and depression, and rapidly fluctuating mood ('rapid cycling'). These differences may be explained by hormonal factors such as changing levels of sex hormones, and women are at a particularly high risk of relapse during the post-partum period (the period after giving birth) when hormonal changes are both rapid and pronounced.

Are all ethnic groups equally affected?

Bipolar disorder appears to be equally common in all races and ethnicities. There is some evidence to suggest that ethnicity might affect the symptom profile, with, for example, African and African–Caribbean groups more likely to suffer a first episode of mania and more likely to experience severe psychotic symptoms. More research is needed in this area, particularly because of its implications for the assessment and treatment of bipolar sufferers from ethnic minorities.

Why does bipolar disorder affect some people and not others?

Genes

Bipolar disorder has a strong genetic basis, stronger than for any other mental illness. First-degree relatives of a person with bipolar disorder such as siblings and sons and daughters have an approximately 10 per cent risk of themselves developing bipolar

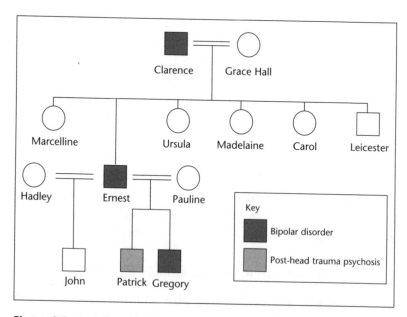

Figure 2.1   Family tree of the famous writer Ernest Hemingway, who suffered from bipolar disorder (adapted from Kay Redfield Jamison (1996), *Touched with Fire: Manic Depressive Illness and the Artistic Temperament*). Bipolar disorder has a strong genetic basis, and both Hemingway's father and his son Gregory had the illness.

disorder in their lifetime, and second-degree relatives such as grandchildren and nephews and nieces have an approximately 4 per cent risk. Both first- and second-degree relatives also have an increased risk of developing other mood disorders such as unipolar depression and schizoaffective disorder, suggesting that there is an overlap in the genes that cause bipolar disorder, unipolar depression, and schizoaffective disorder. The family tree of the writer Ernest Hemingway gives an example of a family with a higher than average incidence of bipolar disorder (see Figure 2.1).

If a person with an identical twin (that is, a twin who shares exactly the same genes) develops bipolar disorder, the chance of the identical twin also developing the illness is about 60 per cent. This is significantly higher than for other mental illnesses such as schizophrenia or depression, and it confirms that genes are a very important factor in the causation of bipolar disorder.

Important as they are, if genes were the only factor involved in the causation of bipolar disorder, then the chance of an identical twin also developing the illness given that his or her twin already has the illness might be expected to be 100 per cent. As this is not the case, other factors must also be involved in the causation of bipolar disorder. These other factors include stress and life events, disturbances in sleep pattern, and drug misuse.

Stress and 'life events'

Although genes play a very important role in the causation of bipolar disorder, there is no single gene that can be said to cause bipolar disorder. Rather, there are several genes that are independent of one another and that, cumulatively, make a person more or less vulnerable to developing the illness, and also to developing other mental illnesses such as depressive disorder and schizoaffective disorder. A person who is highly vulnerable to developing bipolar disorder but who is never subjected to severe stress may never develop the illness. On the other hand, a person who is less vulnerable to developing the illness but who comes under severe stress may develop it. Examples of severe stress include getting divorced, losing a friend or relative in an accident, or suffering from a health or financial crisis. The situation is analogous to that of many other important conditions such as heart disease or diabetes. Taking heart disease as an example, every person inherits a certain complement of genes that make him or her more or less vulnerable to developing the illness. Regardless of this vulnerability, if he or she maintains a healthy diet, takes regular exercise, and drinks in moderation, then he or she is likely to stay healthy or at least to suffer less from the illness.

Thus, a person may develop bipolar disorder if the stress that he or she faces becomes greater than his or her ability to cope with it. This stress is often related to life events – that is, to important events such as those listed above: getting divorced and so on. Though life events need not be negative, they are invariably perceived as being highly stressful. Thus events such as getting married, having a baby, or going on holiday can count as significant life events for certain people. The corollary of this is that life events are subjective: a life event for me is not necessarily a life event for you, and vice versa.

From Figure 2.2 it can be seen that, on the one hand, life events can precipitate the symptoms of bipolar disorder and that, on the other, bipolar disorder can precipitate life events. For example, if a person is suffering from a depressive episode and from difficulty concentrating and lack of energy, he or she is more likely to lose his or her job than the average person. So, as you can see, the relationship between life events and bipolar disorder is far from being a simple one.

Although life events can cause a lot of stress, most of the stress that a person experiences on a daily basis does not come

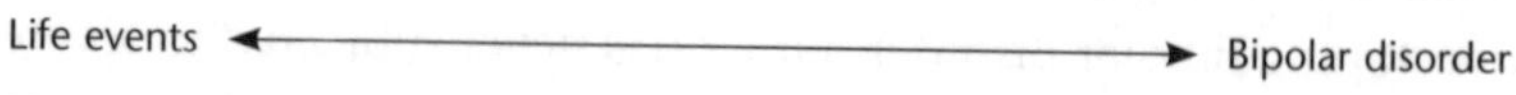

Life events ⟵――――――――――――――――――――→ Bipolar disorder

Figure 2.2 The relationship between life events and bipolar disorder.

from life events, but from seemingly smaller 'background' stressors such as tense relationships, painful memories (especially memories of childhood physical or sexual abuse, loss, or abandonment), isolation, discrimination, poor housing, or unpaid bills. The cumulative effect of these stressors can be far greater than that of any single life event and may alone be sufficient to tip a person into bipolar disorder.

A final point about stress is that different people are able to handle different amounts of it. The amount of stress that a given person is able to handle is related to his or her genetic vulnerability to bipolar disorder, but also to his or her thinking and coping styles and aptitude for social interaction. People with positive coping and thinking styles and good social skills are better able to diffuse stressful situations – for example, by doing something about them, by putting them in their correct context, or simply by talking about them and 'sharing the pain'.

Sleep disturbances

Loss of sleep or irregular sleep patterns can trigger a manic episode in people with bipolar disorder or who are at risk of developing bipolar disorder. Even going to bed unusually late, for example after having to meet an important deadline or after a big night out, can be sufficient to trigger a manic episode. For this reason, people with bipolar disorder who are students at university, who work long hours, or who work shifts are at particular risk of developing a manic episode. People with bipolar disorder may also develop a manic episode after travelling across several time zones and needing to readjust their internal clocks and sleep patterns. If a person's mood becomes even slightly abnormally elevated, he or she may be unable to sleep. As sleep is lost, his or her mood is likely to become even more abnormally elevated. As you can see, a vicious circle quickly takes hold. For the person with bipolar disorder, it is all-important to recognize this vicious circle early and to cut it short (see chapter 10).

Drug and alcohol misuse

Recent research has found that, compared with all people with bipolar disorder, people with bipolar disorder who abuse illicit drugs or alcohol have an earlier onset of illness and a poorer outcome, and are more likely to be admitted to a psychiatric hospital. Stimulant drugs such as amphetamines, ecstasy, and cocaine can trigger a manic episode, whereas alcohol and tranquillizers can trigger a depressive episode.

Some people with bipolar disorder turn to drugs or alcohol to obtain relief from their symptoms and from their legitimate feelings of sadness and anxiety. These drugs may temporarily blunt or mask symptoms, but in the long term they are likely to lead to more frequent and severe relapses of the illness. People who use drugs may also delay getting help, including getting a much-needed prescription for medication.

Medication

A bipolar sufferer with a severe depressive episode may be treated with an antidepressant, but in some cases he or she may be 'over-treated' and end up with a manic episode. This 'manic switch', as it is sometimes called, is an important problem in the management of bipolar disorder. Apart from antidepressants, other medications that can trigger a manic episode include steroids, thyroid medication, appetite suppressants, over-the-counter flu remedies, and caffeine. Medications that can trigger a depressive episode include steroids, beta-blockers, and digoxin.

Seasonal changes

Manic episodes are more common in spring and summer. This is probably explained by seasonal changes in the weather and, in particular, by increases in ambient light. This finding may be at the origin of the expression 'This is very midsummer madness' used by Shakespeare in *Twelfth Night*. In contrast, depressive episodes are more common in autumn and winter.

Season-of-birth effect

Also related to seasonal changes is the finding that people born between the months of January and April are at a slightly higher risk of developing a mood disorder. This higher risk is referred to as the 'season-of-birth effect' and is thought to result from events that take place before the birth or at the time of the birth. An example of such an event is a viral infection in the foetus, which is more common during winter months.

Obstetric complications

There is also some limited evidence to suggest that obstetric complications (complications during pregnancy and at the time of delivery) can increase the risk of a child later developing bipolar disorder.

During pregnancy and the period after giving birth, women with bipolar disorder or at risk of developing bipolar disorder have about twice the risk of developing an episode of elevated or depressed mood. This is in part because many choose to stop their mood-stabilizing medication, because they are concerned about the effects that the medication may have on their unborn or breast-feeding child. At the same time, they recognize that suffering from an episode of mood disorder can have equally serious implications for their child, not to mention themselves. Thus managing bipolar disorder throughout pregnancy involves balancing the risks of the illness with the risks and benefits of its treatment (see chapter 9).

How is the brain affected in bipolar disorder?

The symptoms of mania result from an excess of certain excitatory neurotransmitters, or chemical messengers, in the brain. These neurotransmitters include the monoamines dopamine, noradrenaline, and serotonin. Drugs that increase the release of these neurotransmitters, such as antidepressants or stimulant drugs such as amphetamines and cocaine, can elevate mood. In contrast, the symptoms of depression result from the depletion of these monoamines or from a change in the functioning of their receptors.

In particular, the central role of dopamine over-activity in mania is supported by strong evidence that medication that blocks the dopamine D_2 receptor in the brain is effective in the treatment of mania. That having been said, changes in the activity levels of dopamine and other monoamines in the brain do not provide a complete explanation for the symptoms of manic and depressive episodes, and more research is needed in this area.

In conclusion

It appears that a person's risk of developing bipolar disorder depends largely on his or her genetic make-up. However, this risk may not be actualized unless the person experiences a higher level of stress than he or she can cope with. Stress results from environmental factors and can come in several forms, such as life events, background stress, unhelpful thinking and coping styles, sleep deprivation, and drugs. Stress in any one of those forms may also result in stress in one or several other forms. For example, stress from losing a loved one may lead to sleeplessness, alcohol misuse, and financial difficulties. A vicious circle can take hold, and the cumulative stress becomes sufficient to tip the person into an episode of mood disorder. This pattern helps to explain many episodes of mood disorder, but by no means all; sometimes, an episode of mood disorder may not have any apparent trigger.

3

Symptoms

Case study 1

'I have been high several times over the years, but low only once.

When I was high, I became very enthusiastic about some project or another and would work on it with determination and success. During such highs I wrote the bulk of two books and stood for parliament as an independent. I went to bed very late, if at all, and woke up very early. I didn't feel tired at all. There were times when I lost touch with reality and got carried away. At such times, I would jump from project to project without completing any, and did many things that I later regretted. Once I thought that I was Jesus and that I had a mission to save the world. It was an extremely alarming thought.

When I was low I was an entirely different person. I felt as though life was pointless and that there was nothing worth living for. Although I would not have tried to end my life, I would not have regretted death. I did not have the wish or the energy to do even the simplest of tasks. Instead I withered away my days sleeping or lying awake in bed, worrying about the financial problems that I had created for myself during my highs. I also had a feeling of unreality, that people were conspiring to make life seem normal when in actual fact it was unreal. Several times I asked the doctor and the nurses to show me their ID because I just couldn't bring myself to believe that they were real.'

Case study 2

Ten months ago Mrs S., a community psychiatric nurse, started feeling brighter and more energetic. At work she took on many extra hours and extra roles, but to her surprise one of her colleagues reported her as unsafe. She then resigned, claiming that she needed more time to devote to her plans and projects. By then she couldn't stop her thoughts from racing and was sleeping only three or four hours a night. She rented a launderette and set out to transform it into a multipurpose centre. Then she bought three houses to rent out to the poor. She became very out-going and acted completely out of character, dressing garishly, smoking marijuana, and getting herself arrested for being 'drunk and disorderly'. Four months ago her mood began dropping and she felt dreadful and ashamed. Today she is feeling better but has had to sell her house to pay off her debts. Her psychiatrist suggested that she start on a mood stabilizer, but she is understandably reluctant to take his advice.

What are the symptoms of a manic episode?

Manic episodes usually begin abruptly over a period of days and, without treatment, last for an average of about four months. Depressive episodes usually begin more gradually and, without treatment, last for an average of about six months. They rarely last for more than a year, except in the elderly. In bipolar disorder, the frequency and severity of manic and depressive episodes is very variable, as is the proportion of manic to depressive episodes.

Mania is characterized by persistently elevated, expansive, or irritable mood that is accompanied by some or all of the following:

- Inflated self-esteem or grandiosity
- Pressure of thoughts, or thoughts racing through the mind
- Pressure of speech, or pressure to keep talking
- Increased energy and over-activity
- Decreased need for sleep
- Distractibility
- Disinhibited behaviour that can have painful consequences

The *International Classification of Diseases* (ICD) describes mania thus:

Mood is elevated out of keeping with the individual's circumstances and may vary from carefree joviality to almost uncontrollable excitement. Elation is accompanied by increased energy, resulting in over-activity, pressure of speech, and a decreased need for sleep. Normal social inhibitions are lost, attention cannot be sustained, and there is often marked distractibility. Self-esteem is inflated, and grandiose or over-optimistic ideas are expressed.

Perceptual disorders may occur, such as the appreciation of colours as especially vivid ... The individual may embark on extravagant and impractical schemes, spend money recklessly, or become aggressive, amorous, or facetious in inappropriate circumstances. In some manic episodes the mood is irritable and suspicious rather than elated.

In mania the disturbance in mood is sufficiently severe to cause a marked impairment in occupational or social functioning, and it may require hospitalization to prevent the person from directly or indirectly harming himself or herself, or others. In some cases, psychotic symptoms may be present.

What are psychotic symptoms?

Psychotic symptoms consist of hallucinations and delusions, which are usually as real to the bipolar sufferer as they are unreal to everybody else. They may be experienced both in manic episodes and in severe depressive episodes.

Hallucinations

Psychiatrists define an hallucination as a 'sense perception that arises in the absence of a stimulus'. Hallucinations involve hearing, seeing, smelling, tasting, or feeling things that are not actually there. The most common hallucinations in both mania and depression are auditory hallucinations – hallucinations of sounds and voices. Voices can either speak directly *to* the person with bipolar disorder (second-person – 'you' – voices) or *about* him or her (third-person – 'he' or 'she' – voices). Voices can be highly distressing, especially if they involve threats or abuse, or if they are loud and incessant. Carers might begin to experience something of the distress of hearing voices by turning on both the radio and the television at the same time, both at full volume, and then trying to hold a normal conversation.

Delusions

Delusions are defined as being 'strongly held beliefs that are not amenable to logic or persuasion and that are out of keeping with their holder's background'. Although delusions are not necessarily false, the process by which they are arrived at is bizarre and illogical. In mania, the delusions are usually 'mood-congruent' – that is, in keeping with the elevated mood – and may involve delusions of being invested with special status, a special purpose, or special abilities – for example, being the most intelligent person on earth and having the responsibility of saving it from the effects of climate change. Sometimes, there may also be delusions of being persecuted (even by loved ones), of being talked about or referred to (for example, on public transport or on the TV or radio), or of having one's thoughts, actions, and bodily functions controlled by an outside force.

Are people with psychotic symptoms dangerous or unpredictable?

Psychotic symptoms correspond closely to the general public's idea of 'madness', and so people with prominent psychotic symptoms may evoke feelings of fear and anxiety in others. Such feelings are often reinforced by selective reporting in the media of the rare headline tragedies involving people with (usually untreated) mental illness. The reality is that the vast majority of people with bipolar disorder are no more likely than the average person to pose a risk to others, but far more likely than the average person to pose a risk to themselves. For example, they may neglect their safety and personal care, or may leave themselves open to being emotionally, physically, or financially exploited by others.

How can carers manage psychotic symptoms?

Psychotic symptoms can be particularly distressing, both to the person with bipolar disorder and to his or her carers. Carers often find themselves challenging the hallucinations and delusions, partly out of a desire to be helpful, and partly out of understandable feelings of fear and helplessness. Unfortunately this can be counterproductive, since it can alienate the person with bipolar disorder from his or her carers at the very time that he or she needs them the most. Although it can be difficult, carers should try to remember that psychotic symptoms are as real to the person having them as they are unreal to everybody else.

So, a more helpful course of action for carers is to recognize that hallucinations and delusions are real and important to the person having them while making it clear that they do not personally share in them. For example:

PERSON: An archangel told me that I am the chosen one, and that my mission is to go forth and save mankind from sin.

CARER: Are you hearing him now?

PERSON: No, he's just stopped talking.

CARER: What else did he say?

PERSON: That to succeed I must fight with the devil.

CARER: That sounds terribly frightening.

PERSON: I've never felt so frightened in my life.

CARER: I can understand that you feel frightened, although I myself have never heard this archangel you speak about.

PERSON: You mean, you've never heard him?

CARER: No, not at all.

PERSON: What about the devil? Have you heard him?

CARER: No, I haven't heard him either. Have you tried ignoring these voices?

PERSON: If I listen to my iPod then they don't seem so loud, and I don't feel so frightened.

CARER: What about when we talk together, like now?

PERSON: That's very helpful too.

What is it like to meet a person with mania?

People with mania may be dressed in colourful clothing or in unusual combinations of clothing. They may be wearing an excessive number of inappropriate accessories, or excessive make-up, jewellery, or body art. Their behaviour is typically hyperactive, and they may be entertaining, flirtatious, vigilant, assertive, or aggressive, and sometimes all of these in turn. While they are typically euphoric, optimistic, self-confident, and grandiose, they may also be irritable or tearful, with rapid and unexpected shifts from one extreme to the other. They may feel that their thoughts are racing, and as a result they may speak very fast and feel pressured to keep on talking. Sometimes they may have difficulty getting to the point, or may coin new words and talk in rhymes and puns. All this can make it very difficult for others to be heard, and people with mania may not be able to concentrate on what people around them are saying. They are typically full of grandiose and unrealistic plans that they begin acting upon but then soon abandon. They also often engage in pleasure-seeking, risk-taking, impulsive, and disin-hibited behaviour, which may for example involve taking illegal drugs, engaging in sexual activity with near-strangers, driving recklessly and endangering lives, or spending vast amounts of money with careless abandon. Such behaviour may damage their physical health, leave them open to exploitation, or land them in trouble with the police and authorities. People with mania can also experience psychotic symptoms such as hallu-cinations or delusions that make their behaviour all the more difficult to explain. Insight into the illness is often very poor, and they typically find it very difficult to accept that they are ill. As a result, great damage can be done to relationships, jobs, careers, finances, and health.

What are the symptoms of a hypomanic episode?

Hypomania is a lesser degree of mania, with similar symptoms to those of mania but less severe or extreme. The mood is ele-vated, expansive, or irritable but, in contrast to mania, there are no psychotic features and no *marked* impairment of social functioning. Indeed, some people with hypomania may function very effectively, be full of ideas and energy, and be the 'life and soul' of the party. Nevertheless, they often lack judgement and so make rash and damaging or dangerous decisions. Hypomania may herald mania and, in such cases, the diagnosis should be one of mania only.

What are the symptoms of a depressive episode?

William Styron, the author of *Sophie's Choice* and other novels, wrote a book called *Darkness Visible* about his experience of being depressed. This is a particularly poignant extract from the book:

> In depression this faith in deliverance, in ultimate restoration is absent. The pain is unrelenting, and what makes the condition intolerable is the foreknowledge that no remedy will come – not in a day, an hour, a month, or a minute. If there is mild relief, one knows that it is only temporary; more pain will follow. It is hopelessness even more than pain that crushes the soul. So the decision-making of daily life involves not, as in normal affairs, shifting from one annoying situation to another less annoying – or from discomfort to relative comfort, or from boredom to activity – but moving from pain to pain. One does not abandon, even briefly, one's bed of nails, but is attached to it wherever one goes.

The symptoms of depression are listed in Table 3.1.

Although the most common symptom of depression is depressed mood or sadness, many people with depression do not complain of this, and instead complain of psychological or biological symptoms that prevent them from fulfilling their social obligations. For example, they may complain of feeling tired all the time, or find that they cannot concentrate on their job or that they can no longer care for their children.

People with only mild depression often complain of feeling depressed and tired all the time, and sometimes also complain of

Table 3.1 Symptoms of depression

Core symptoms of depression
Sadness
Lack of interest and enjoyment
Feeling tired easily
Psychological symptoms of depression
Poor concentration
Poor motivation and energy
Poor self-esteem and self-confidence
Feelings of guilt
Pessimistic outlook
Biological features of depression
Sleep disturbance – for example, waking up early in the morning
Loss of appetite or weight loss (or both)
Loss of libido
Retardation (slowing down) of speech and movements

feeling stressed or anxious. There are none of the biological symptoms of depression such as sleep disturbance, loss of appetite, and retardation of speech and movements and, although suicidal thoughts can occur, they are only uncommonly acted upon.

People with moderate depression present with many if not most of the symptoms listed in Table 3.1. These symptoms are present to such an intense degree that they find fulfilling their social obligations difficult. Biological symptoms and anhedonia (the loss of the capacity to experience pleasure from previously pleasurable experiences) are characteristic. Suicidal ideation is common and may be acted upon.

People with severe depression essentially have an exaggerated form of moderate depression, typically with intense negative feelings and prominent retardation of movements. Suicidal risk is high. Psychotic symptoms may be present and are usually mood-congruent – that is, in keeping with the depressed mood;

for example, there may be delusions of guilt, nihilistic delusions, or somatic delusions. Delusions of guilt are delusions of having committed a crime or of having sinned greatly – for example, being personally responsible for a recent earthquake or terrorist attack and therefore deserving of severe punishment. Nihilistic delusions are delusions that one no longer exists or that one is about to die or suffer a personal catastrophe. In some cases there may be a belief that other people or objects no longer exist or that the world is coming to an end. Somatic delusions, sometimes also called hypochondriacal delusions, are delusions of being physically ill or having deformed body parts. These delusional themes can present alone or in combination, and they are often elaborated upon – that is, developed into a complex system of delusional beliefs.

What is a mixed episode?

A mixed episode, sometimes also called a mixed state, is an episode of mood disorder in which there are prominent symptoms of both mania and depression at the same time. This may, for example, involve tearfulness during a manic episode or racing thoughts during a depressive episode. This combination of manic activation and depressed mood is sometimes referred to as 'agitated depression', which predisposes to illicit drug misuse and attempted suicide.

What is rapid cycling?

'Rapid cycling' affects about one in six people with bipolar disorder. It refers to four or more episodes of mania, hypomania, depression, or mixed states in a period of one year. A person with rapid cycling may go from one episode of mood disorder to the next without experiencing a period of normal mood in between. Rapid cycling can be induced or exacerbated by antidepressants, especially if the person is not also on a mood stabilizer.

4

Diagnosis

The majority of medical conditions are defined either by their cause ('aetiology') or by the damage to the body ('pathology') that they result from, and for this reason are relatively easy to define and recognize. For example, malaria is caused by protozoan parasites of the genus *Plasmodium*, and cerebral infarction ('stroke') results from the obstruction of an artery in the brain. Unfortunately mood disorders, in common with most mental illnesses, cannot as yet be defined by their aetiology and pathology, and so must be defined according to their clinical manifestations or symptoms. Thus, a psychiatrist must base a diagnosis of mood disorder solely on the symptoms manifested by his or her patient, without the help of either blood tests (as in malaria) or brain scans (as in stroke).

To do this, the psychiatrist must rely on clearly defined concepts and reliable operational criteria. These are provided in classifications of mental illness, and particularly in ICD-10 and DSM-IV. The *ICD-10 Classification of Mental and Behavioural Disorders: clinical descriptions and diagnostic guidelines*, published in 1992, is chapter V of the *Tenth Revision of the International Classification of Diseases* (ICD-10). Unlike the other chapters, which simply list and code the names of diseases and disorders, chapter V also provides clinical descriptions and diagnostic criteria. These are based on scientific literature and international consultation and consensus, because ICD-10 is for use in all countries. The fourth revision of the *Diagnostic and Statistical Manual of Mental Disorders* (DSM-IV), first published in 1994 by the American Psychiatric Association, is an alternative but influential classification that is nonetheless broadly similar to the ICD-10 classification.

How are mood disorders classified?

A scheme of the various types of mood disorder is shown in Figure 4.1 (overleaf).

Primary versus secondary mood disorders

Disorders of mood can be either *primary* or *secondary*. A primary mood disorder is one which does *not* result from another medical or psychiatric condition. A secondary (or 'organic') mood disorder, on the other hand, is one that *does* result from another medical or psychiatric condition (for example, from anaemia, hypothyroidism, or agoraphobia, or as a result of alcohol or drug misuse). If your family doctor or psychiatrist makes a diagnosis of a mood disorder, he or she carefully considers the possibility that it might be a secondary mood disorder, because a secondary mood disorder is often most effectively treated by treating the primary condition that gave rise to it – the anaemia or hypothyroidism, for example.

Unipolar disorder versus bipolar disorder

Broadly speaking, a primary mood disorder is either unipolar (depressive disorder, dysthymia) or bipolar (bipolar affective disorder, cyclothymia). To meet the criteria for a bipolar mood disorder, a person must have had one or more episodes of mania or hypomania. The unipolar–bipolar distinction is an important one to make, because the course and treatment of bipolar disorder differ significantly from those of unipolar depression.

Unipolar mood disorders

In ICD-10, depressive disorders are classified according to their severity into mild, moderate, severe, and psychotic depressive disorder. If a patient has had more than one episode of depressive disorder, the term 'recurrent depressive disorder' is used, and the current episode is classified as for a single episode (for example, 'recurrent depressive disorder, current episode moderate').

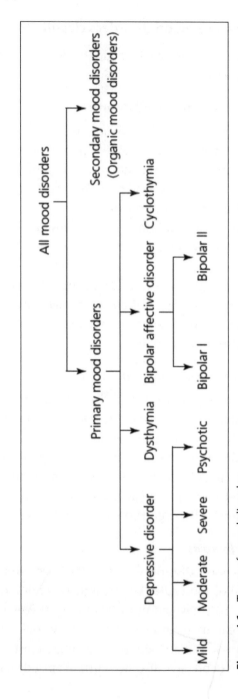

Figure 4.1 Types of mood disorder.

In DSM-IV, the term 'major depression' is used instead of depressive disorder. Major depression is classified simply as 'single episode' or 'recurrent'.

Not all people suffering from depressive symptoms have a depressive disorder. Dysthymia is characterized by depressive symptoms that are not sufficiently severe to meet a diagnosis of depressive disorder. Although dysthymia has sometimes been regarded as a 'depressive personality', genetic studies suggest that it is in fact a chronic (that is, long-term) and mild form of depression (see Figure 4.2).

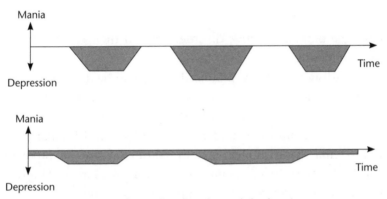

Figure 4.2 Recurrent depressive disorder and dysthymia.

Bipolar mood disorders

According to ICD-10, 'bipolar affective disorder' consists of repeated (two or more) episodes of depression and mania or hypomania. In the absence of episodes of mania or hypomania, the diagnosis is one of recurrent depressive disorder. In the absence of episodes of depression, the diagnosis is one of bipolar affective disorder (in other words, recurrent episodes of mania are diagnosed as bipolar affective disorder). This is not only because sooner or later a depressive episode is almost certain to supervene, but also because recurrent episodes of mania

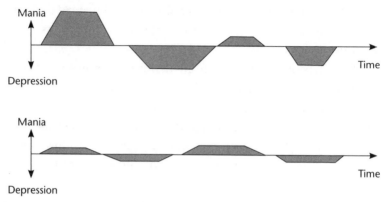

Figure 4.3   Type I bipolar disorder and cyclothymia.

resemble bipolar affective disorder both in their course and in their outcome.

According to DSM-IV, bipolar disorder can be diagnosed after even a single episode of mania, whereas in ICD-10 a single episode of mania is simply diagnosed as a 'manic episode'. The separation of bipolar disorder into bipolar I and bipolar II in DSM-IV may have implications for treatment response. Bipolar I consists of episodes of mania and major depression, and bipolar II of episodes of hypomania and major depression.

Cyclothymia can be described as mild chronic (or long-term) bipolar disorder and is characterized by numerous episodes of mild elation and mild depressive symptoms that are not sufficiently severe or prolonged to meet the criteria for bipolar disorder or recurrent depressive disorder. Cyclothymia is compared graphically with type I bipolar disorder in Figure 4.3.

How is a diagnosis of bipolar disorder made?

If a person is suspected of having malaria, a blood sample can be taken and examined under a microscope for malarial parasites. Similarly, if a person is suspected of having an abnormal rhythm of the heart, a heart tracing can be recorded so that the abnormal rhythm can be identified. On the other hand, if a person is suspected of having bipolar disorder, there are no laboratory or physical tests that can confirm the diagnosis. Instead, the psychiatrist must base his or her diagnosis on the person's symptoms. These must meet certain agreed criteria listed in diagnostic manuals such as ICD-10 and DSM-IV. For a manic episode to be diagnosed, the DSM-IV criteria are approximately as follows.

First, there should be a period of abnormally and persistently elevated, expansive, or irritable mood lasting for at least one week or any duration if hospitalization is necessary.

Second, during this period of mood disturbance, at least three of the following symptoms should have been present to a significant degree:

- Inflated self-esteem or grandiosity
- Decreased need for sleep
- More talkative than usual or pressure to keep talking
- Flight of ideas, that is, subjective experiences that thoughts are racing
- Distractibility
- Agitation or increase in goal-directed activity
- Involvement in pleasurable activities that can have painful consequences

Third, the symptoms should not meet criteria for a mixed episode.

Fourth, the mood disturbance should be sufficiently severe to cause marked impairment in occupational or social functioning or to require hospitalization or be accompanied by psychotic features.

Fifth, the symptoms should not be due to a substance or a general medical condition.

Table 4.1   Conditions that can present like bipolar disorder (mania)

Psychiatric conditions

Drug use – for example, alcohol, amphetamines, ecstasy, cocaine

Schizophrenia

Schizoaffective disorder: more or less equally prominent symptoms of both schizophrenia and mood disorder (depression or mania)

Severe depression with psychotic symptoms

Other psychotic disorders – for example, brief psychotic disorder, a condition that resembles schizophrenia but is relatively short-lived

Cyclothymia: recurrent episodes of mild elation and mild depressive symptoms that are not sufficiently severe or prolonged to meet the diagnostic criteria for bipolar disorder; can be thought of as a mild form of bipolar disorder

Personality disorder

Attention-deficit hyperactivity disorder: difficulty maintaining attention and over-activity that can persist into adulthood

Medical conditions

Organic brain disease of the frontal lobes – for example, stroke, multiple sclerosis, brain tumours, epilepsy, AIDS, neurosyphilis

Infectious diseases affecting the brain

Head injury

Endocrine disorders – for example, hyperthyroidism, Cushing's syndrome

Systemic lupus erythematosus

Sleep deprivation

Medications such as antidepressants, steroids, and L-dopa

How long does it take to make a diagnosis of bipolar disorder?

The psychiatrist sets about excluding psychiatric and medical conditions that can present like bipolar disorder (see Table 4.1) by obtaining a clear and detailed picture of the person's symptoms and his or her personal and family history, usually over a protracted period of time. During this time, he or she may also conduct a full physical examination, obtain blood and urine samples, and arrange for a brain scan such as a computed tomography (CT) scan or a magnetic resonance imaging (MRI) scan. In some cases, he or she may arrange for a second psychiatrist or other specialist (such as a neurologist or endocrinologist) to provide a second opinion. Only after the psychiatrist has confidently ruled out other psychiatric and medical conditions can a firm diagnosis of bipolar disorder be made.

When should help be sought?

There is reliable scientific evidence that early detection and intervention in bipolar disorder improves outcomes. Many people with bipolar disorder remain undiagnosed for a long period of time, perhaps several years. This may be for one of several reasons:

- They may have only manic or hypomanic episodes, during which they feel good and full of energy, and therefore see no reason to seek treatment.
- They may so far have had only depressive episodes, and have therefore been given a diagnosis of recurrent depressive disorder.
- Their symptoms may have suggested another, incorrect diagnosis, such as schizophrenia or schizoaffective disorder.
- They may fear the stigma of mental illness and so are reluctant to seek out the help that they need.

Early detection and intervention in bipolar disorder improves outcomes, not only by shortening the ongoing episode of mood disorder, but also by minimizing the risks of further episodes of mood disorder. This in turn minimizes the risk of complications such as broken careers and relationships, alcohol and drug misuse, and suicide.

5

Coping with a diagnosis of bipolar disorder

A diagnosis of bipolar disorder can be difficult to accept, both for the person diagnosed and for his or her relatives. Like heart disease or diabetes, bipolar disorder is a serious and potentially debilitating illness. But unlike heart disease or diabetes, bipolar disorder is poorly understood and is stigmatized by the general public. This is in no small part due to sensationalist reporting in the media of violent acts committed by a very small number of people with psychotic illnesses. The reality is, of course, that bipolar disorder is a common illness that can be effectively treated and that only rarely results in people becoming dangerous.

Owing to the stigma attached to a diagnosis of bipolar disorder, some people may decide or be persuaded to consult a second or third psychiatrist – often at large expense – in the hope of having the diagnosis changed or reversed. Others may simply deny the diagnosis, and instead refer to their illness according to labels that they consider to be less stigmatizing, such as depression or an anxiety disorder. Some people may even prefer to tell others that they are in hospital because they have a brain tumour or because they are in a drug rehabilitation programme. Other people, particularly those suffering from prominent psychotic symptoms, such as delusions or hallucinations, may altogether deny that they are ill. This may be because of the stigma attached to bipolar disorder, but also because their delusions and hallucinations seem perfectly real to them, or because they actually feel good and full of energy.

In contrast, some people experience a great sense of relief at being given a diagnosis of bipolar disorder, because it enables them to get the help that they need and to make the fastest and most complete recovery possible.

Unlike illnesses such as heart disease or diabetes, bipolar disorder tends to strike in the prime of life, when people are likely to be full of plans and dreams for the future. In some cases, they may feel under intense pressure to succeed and be successful. As a result of being given a diagnosis of bipolar disorder, people may feel that all their dreams have been shattered and that they have betrayed those that they hold most near and dear. Mixed feelings of loss, hopelessness, and guilt may exacerbate or prolong a depressive episode or give rise to further depressive episodes and, in some cases, even to thoughts of self-harm or suicide. In such cases, it is important to remember that increasing numbers of people with bipolar disorder make a durable recovery and that many others are able to lead productive and fulfilling lives. Indeed, some bipolar sufferers such as Stephen Fry, Mark Twain, and Robert Lowell and many others have even gone on to make unique and important contributions to society. Virginia Woolf, the novelist and member of the Bloomsbury group, wrote about her experience of bipolar disorder thus:

> I married, and then my brains went up like a shower of fireworks. As an experience, madness is terrific I can assure you, and not to be sniffed at; and in its lava I still find most of the things I write about. It shoots out of one everything shaped, final, not in mere driblets as sanity does. And the six months ... that I lay in bed taught me a good deal about what is called oneself.
>
> Quoted from a letter by Virginia Woolf to her friend
> Ethel Smyth

You can make the future yours again, as you are doing by making the effort to read this book.

Finally, remember: you are not to blame for your illness, and you must not think that you have done anything to 'deserve' it. Do not let your parents blame themselves for your illness either.

Just like anybody else, people with bipolar disorder can have good parents, bad parents, and absent parents. Far from being to blame, parents are often their child's most valuable source of structure and support and their greatest hope for a permanent recovery. Bipolar disorder is a common illness that is in large part genetically determined. It is not anybody's fault.

Many bipolar sufferers find it difficult to accept that they are mentally ill, and as a result they can be reluctant to help themselves or accept help from others. Bipolar disorder is a serious illness and leaving it untreated can have grave consequences for your short-term and long-term mental and physical health. The fear and isolation, not to mention the effects of the illness itself, can lead to a vicious circle of hopelessness, neglect, and alcohol and drug misuse. By accepting your psychiatrist's diagnosis, talking about it, reading about it, and seeking the help that you need, you are taking personal control over your illness and giving yourself the best chances of a long-term recovery. Remember that you are not alone, and that many people have once faced a similar situation. Talking to these people can provide you with much-needed information and support, and help to alleviate any feelings of fear and isolation that you may have.

Will I get better?

Without treatment, manic episodes last for an average duration of about four months and depressive episodes last for an average duration of about six months. The frequency and severity of manic and depressive episodes is very variable, as is the proportion of manic to depressive episodes. After a first manic episode, as many as 90 per cent or nine in ten of all people with bipolar disorder experience further manic or depressive episodes. In many cases, the interval between episodes gets progressively shorter, particularly if the person is not receiving adequate treatment with mood-stabilizing medication. The outlook is particularly bad in rapid-cycling bipolar disorder, but relatively good in bipolar II, which is the form of bipolar disorder that involves episodes of depression and hypomania, rather than depression and mania (see Chapter 4). On average, a person with bipolar disorder can expect to suffer a total of between eight and ten episodes of either mania or depression during the course of his or her lifetime, but this is only an average and the number of episodes suffered varies a lot from one person to another.

Sadly, about 10 per cent of people with bipolar disorder eventually commit suicide, and the rate of attempted suicide (unsuccessful suicide attempts) and self-harm is higher still. The risk of suicide is highest during episodes of depression and mixed episodes involving symptoms of both mania and depression. Factors that are likely to increase the risk of suicide include being male, being young, being unmarried, lacking social support, having high intelligence, having high ambitions or expectations, being early in the course of the illness, having good insight into the illness, and being recently discharged from a psychiatric hospital. Accidents are also common, particularly during manic episodes when behaviour can be impulsive, disinhibited, and reckless. For example, people with bipolar disorder may suffer from an accidental drug overdose, car crash, house fire, or unplanned pregnancy. People with bipolar disorder may also suffer from neglect (for example, from not eating or drinking).

Virginia Woolf herself committed suicide at the age of 59 by walking into the River Ouse with a large rock in her pocket (as portrayed in *The Hours*, a film loosely based on her novel *Mrs Dalloway* and starring Nicole Kidman as Virginia Woolf). This is her suicide letter to her husband and carer Leonard Woolf:

> Dearest, I feel certain that I am going mad again. I feel we can't go through another of those terrible times. And I shan't recover this time. I begin to hear voices, and I can't concentrate. So I am doing what seems to be the best thing to do. You have given me

the greatest possible happiness. You have been in every way all that anyone could be. I don't think two people could have been happier till this terrible disease came. I can't fight any longer. I know that I am spoiling your life, and that without me you could work. And you will I know. You see I can't even write this properly. I can't read. What I want to say is I owe all the happiness of my life to you. You have been entirely patient with me and incredibly good. I want to say that – everybody knows it. If anybody could have saved me it would have been you. Everything has gone from me but the certainty of your goodness. I can't go on spoiling your life any longer. I don't think two people could have been happier than we have been.

    V.

Life expectancy in bipolar disorder is variable, and depends on the course of the illness and the extent of the recovery made. Overall, the life expectancy of people with bipolar disorder is reduced by about eight to ten years compared with the average life expectancy of the population at large. But this gap is closing as a result of more effective treatments and higher standards of physical care. Cardiovascular diseases are a common cause of death in people with bipolar disorder, but they can be prevented through a healthy diet and regular exercise. One of the most important contributors to cardiovascular diseases in people with bipolar disorder is smoking, so stopping smoking can do much to increase life expectancy. Other common causes of death in bipolar disorder are suicide and self-harm, accidents, and drug overdoses. However, it is important to note that bipolar sufferers who receive treatment and make a good response to treatment make considerably better outcomes than the average bipolar sufferer.

Your individual chances of getting better are difficult to predict, but certain factors about the severity of your illness and your personal circumstances can act as 'positive prognostic factors' – factors that make a positive prognosis (or outcome) more likely. Positive and negative prognostic factors in bipolar disorder are listed in Table 5.1. There are some prognostic factors, such as family history or sex, that cannot be changed,

Table 5.1   Positive and negative prognostic factors in bipolar disorder

Positive prognostic factors	Negative prognostic factors
Lack of a family history	Strong family history
Female sex	Male sex
Onset at an older age	Onset at a younger age
Clear precipitating factors	Absence of clear precipitating factors
Absence of a personality disorder	Presence of a personality disorder
Absence of an anxiety disorder	Presence of an anxiety disorder
No alcohol or drug misuse	Frequent alcohol and drug misuse
Regular sleep patterns	Irregular sleep patterns
Good occupational and social functioning	Poor occupational and social functioning
Good social support	Poor social support
Being married or in a relationship	Being single, separated, or divorced
Receiving early treatment	Delaying treatment
Making a good response to treatment	Making a poor response to treatment
Remaining on long-term treatment	Stopping antipsychotic medication

but there are also many, such as receiving early treatment and remaining on mood-stabilizing medication, that are within your personal control. *Some of the most important things that you can do to put all the chances on your side are to begin treatment early, to remain on treatment for the long-term, to stay off alcohol and drugs, to maintain a regular pattern of sleep, and to remain in good physical health by having a sensible diet and taking regular exercise.*

Bipolar disorder can impair cognitive or intellectual function, and people with bipolar disorder may have problems with short-term and long-term memory and speed of information processing. Such problems become pronounced during episodes of mood disorder, but they may also be evident at other times and may make it more difficult for the person to comply with his or her medication and fully engage with his or her treatment plan. If this is the case for you, you should discuss it with a member of your mental health care team.

6

Mental health-care services

The development of community care

Some 40 or 50 years ago, many if not most people with a first episode of mania or depression would have been admitted to a psychiatric hospital for assessment and treatment, and some may have remained as in-patients for an indefinitely long period of time. In the 1950s and 1960s this so-called institutional model of psychiatric care came under heavy criticism for isolating and institutionalizing people with mental illness and thereby condoning their stigmatization by 'mainstream' society. This led to a trend of removing people with mental illness from psychiatric hospitals, in the hope of integrating them into the community. This trend, greatly facilitated by the advent of the first psychotropic drugs in the 1950s and 1960s, continued throughout the 1970s and 1980s.

In the 1980s, such 'community care' came under heavy criticism after a series of headline-grabbing killings by people with mental illness (in particular with schizophrenia, which is another psychotic disorder). Although acts of violence by people with mental illness are rare, they tend to be sensationally reported in the press, leading to the false impression that this group of people are especially dangerous and unpredictable. The truth is of course very different: people with mental illness are sensitive and vulnerable, and in great need of care and understanding. A small minority may pose a risk, but this risk is far more often to themselves than to others.

Heavy criticism of community care in the 1980s prompted a government inquiry that culminated in the Community Care

Act of 1990, a major piece of legislation that is at the origins of the present, more 'fail-safe' model of community care. According to this model, prior to discharge from a psychiatric hospital each patient should have an agreed care plan, and can, in a minority of cases, be placed on a community supervision order (referred to as a 'supervised discharge').

The advantages of community care are clear. By shifting the emphasis from a person's mental illness to his or her strengths and life aspirations, community care promotes independence and self-reliance, while discouraging isolation and institutionalization and reducing stigmatization. That having been said, a lack of mental health staff and resources can in some cases shift the burden of care onto informal carers, such as relatives and friends, and make it especially difficult to care for those most in need, such as the isolated or the homeless. The advantages and disadvantages of community care are listed in Table 6.1.

Table 6.1   Advantages and disadvantages of community care

Advantages	Disadvantages
By focusing on strengths and life aspirations rather than on psychiatric problems, promotes independence and self-reliance	Lack of staff and resources can place a heavy burden on carers
	Makes it difficult to provide care for those most in need, such as the homeless
Discourages isolation and institutionalization	
	Results in a shortage of hospital beds as scarce resources are diverted to community services
Promotes relapse prevention	
Reduces the stigma of mental illness	In some cases, results in the mentally ill becoming homeless or being housed in the prison service rather than in hospitals
Originally thought to be cheaper than in-patient care, but this notion has recently been challenged	
	Poses a (largely perceived) threat to the safety of the person and of the community

One flew over the cuckoo's nest

Vintery, mintery, cutery, corn,
Apple seed and apple thorn;
Wire, briar, limber lock,
Three geese in a flock.
One flew east,
And one flew west,
And one flew over the cuckoo's nest.

Popular nursery rhyme

The film *One Flew Over the Cuckoo's Nest*, adapted from Ken Kesey's popular 1962 novel of the same name, was directed by Milos Forman and starred Jack Nicholson as the spirited R. P. McMurphy – 'Mac' – and Louise Fletcher as the chilly but softly spoken Nurse Ratched. When Mac arrives at the state mental hospital in Oregon, he challenges the stultifying routine and bureaucratic authoritarianism personified by Nurse Ratched, and pays the price by being drugged, electro-shocked, and, ultimately, lobotomized. Nominated for nine Academy Awards, the film is not only a (belated and contentious) criticism of the institutional model of psychiatric care, but also a metaphor of total institutions – that is, institutions that repress individuality to create a compliant society. It is such criticism of the institutional model of psychiatric care that, in the UK and other countries, led to the development of community care.

Organization of mental health-care services

General practice and Accident and Emergency

If a person is suffering from symptoms similar to those seen in either mania or depression, the first port of call is usually the family doctor or general practitioner (GP). If the GP forms an opinion that a person might be suffering from bipolar disorder or another psychotic illness, he or she is most likely to refer the person to specialist services – either to their local Community Mental Health Team (CMHT) or, in an emergency, to the Crisis Resolution and Home Treatment Team (CRHT).

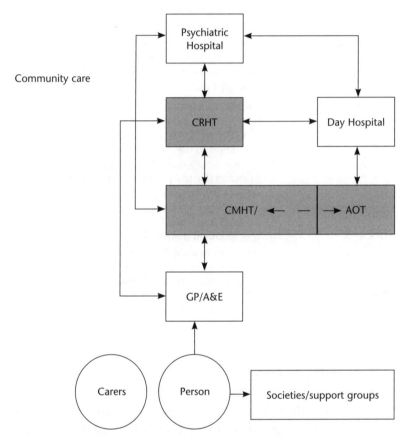

Figure 6.1   Example of organization of mental health-care services (your local services may differ). Note that mental health-care services are organized to facilitate community care and avoid unnecessary hospital admissions. All terms used in this figure are explained in this chapter. CRHT, Crisis Resolution and Home Treatment Team; CMHT, Community Mental Health Team; EIS, Early Intervention Services; AOT or AORT, Assertive Outreach Team; GP, general practitioner (or family doctor); A & E, Accident and Emergency Department.

Table 6.2 Key members of the Community Mental Health Team

Psychiatrist	The psychiatrist is a medical doctor who specializes in diagnosing and treating mental illnesses, such as bipolar disorder, depressive disorders, schizophrenia, and anxiety disorders. The psychiatrist takes a leading role in diagnosing mental illness and formulating a treatment plan
Community psychiatric nurse (CPN)	The CPN is the member of the team that the person with bipolar disorder is likely to come into contact with most often. The CPN usually visits him or her to monitor progress and facilitate the treatment plan
Social worker	Sometimes a person with bipolar disorder may be allocated a social worker instead of or as well as a CPN, in which case the social worker fulfils a role similar to that of the CPN. The social worker can also help to sort out housing and benefits and to ensure that the person makes the most of any services and facilities that are available
Clinical psychologist	'Psychologist' is often confused with 'psychiatrist'. Whereas a psychiatrist is a medical doctor specializing in the diagnosis and treatment of mental illnesses, a psychologist has expertise in the areas of human experience and behaviour. A psychologist may spend time listening to and

A minority of people with symptoms of either mania or depression first present to Accident and Emergency (A and E) rather than to their GP. In this case they are usually screened by a casualty doctor, and then referred for further assessment by a psychiatrist. Again, if the psychiatrist forms an opinion that a person might be suffering from bipolar disorder or another psychotic illness, he or she is most likely to refer the person to their local CMHT or, in an emergency, to the CRHT.

The organization of mental health-care services is illustrated in Figure 6.1.

Table 6.2   cont'd

Clinical psychologist (cont'd)	trying to understand the person with bipolar disorder and his or her carers. A psychologist may also carry out talking therapies such as cognitive–behavioural therapy (see Chapter 8)
Occupational therapist	The role of the occupational therapist is to help the person with bipolar disorder to maintain skills as well as to develop new ones. This not only helps the person to get back to work, but also keeps him or her engaged and motivated. Unfortunately, owing to limited resources, many people with bipolar disorder are not allocated an occupational therapist
Pharmacist	People with bipolar disorder who also have a physical illness or who are pregnant or breast-feeding may find it particularly useful to speak to a pharmacist, who can help with information about medication
Administrative staff	Administrative staff are responsible for arranging appointments and serve as a crucial point of contact both for people with bipolar disorder and their carers and for other members of the team

Note that other forms of support that are available but that do not form part of the CMHT include support groups, telephone help-lines (see Useful addresses), and the Citizens Advice Bureau.

Community Mental Health Team and Assertive Outreach Team

The CMHT is at the centre of mental health-care provision. It is a multidisciplinary team led by a consultant psychiatrist and operating from a team base close to the patients that it serves. Community psychiatric nurses (CPNs) and social workers are key members of the CMHT, often taking a lead in implementing and co-ordinating a person's care and treatment plan and monitoring his or her progress in the community. Other important members of the CMHT include psychiatrists, clinical psychologists, occupational therapists, pharmacists, and administrative staff (see Table 6.2). If a person is referred to a CMHT, he or she usually undergoes an initial assessment by a psychiatrist, sometimes in the presence of another member of the team, such as a CPN or social worker. The skill mix of the multidisciplinary team means that the different parts of the person's life can be understood – and addressed – from a number of different angles.

Some people are reluctant to seek help and treatment, and as a consequence appear at the CMHT only in times of crisis. Paradoxically, these people often have the most complex mental health needs and social problems. For this reason, the responsibility for their care is sometimes transferred to the Assertive Outreach Team (AOT), a specialized multidisciplinary team dedicated to engaging them in treatment and supporting them in their daily activities.

Early Intervention Service

Like the AOT, the Early Intervention Service (EIS) may also operate from the CMHT base. Its role is specifically to improve the short-term and long-term outcomes of schizophrenia and other psychotic illnesses through a three-pronged approach involving preventative measures, earlier detection of untreated cases, and intensive treatment and support at the beginning of the illness.

Crisis Resolution and Home Treatment Team

The Crisis Resolution and Home Treatment Team (CRHT), or 'crisis team' for short, is a 24-hours-a-day, 365-days-a-year multidisciplinary team that in some services acts as a gatekeeper to a variety of psychiatric services, including admission to a psychiatric hospital. People with acute mental health problems are referred to the CRHT from a variety of places and agencies, most commonly GPs, A and E, and CMHTs. A member of the team (often a community psychiatric nurse) promptly assesses the person in conjunction with a psychiatrist to determine if

Table 6.3   Key features of the Crisis Resolution and Home Treatment Team

Gatekeeper to psychiatric services, including admission to a psychiatric hospital
Prompt assessment of patients in a crisis
Intensive, community-based, round-the-clock support in the early stages of the crisis
Continued involvement until the crisis has resolved
Action to prevent similar crises occurring again
Partnership with the person with bipolar disorder and his or her relatives and carers

a hospital admission can be avoided by providing short-term intensive home care. If so, the CRHT arranges for a member of the team to visit the person's home up to three times a day, gradually decreasing the frequency of visits as the person gets better. Other than simply providing support, the CRHT can assist in implementing a care and treatment plan and in monitoring progress. If a person has already been admitted to hospital, the CRHT can also be involved in expediting and facilitating his or her discharge back into the community. The key features of the CRHT are summarized in Table 6.3.

Psychiatric hospital and day hospital

Under the current model of community care, the vast majority of people with a first or subsequent episode of a mood or psychotic disorder are treated in the community. If someone is admitted to hospital this is usually because care in the community is not an option. Possible reasons for admission to a psychiatric hospital are summarized in Table 6.4.

Of the small minority of people with a mood disorder who need to be admitted to a psychiatric hospital, the majority are admitted on a voluntary basis. This is either because they are happy to take the advice of their psychiatrist or carers or because they are frightened of their symptoms and have found

Table 6.4 Possible reasons for admission to a psychiatric hospital

Safety of the person with bipolar disorder, his or her carers, or the general public
Management of acute exacerbations – for example, severe psychotic symptoms
Management of physical complications
Stabilization of medication
Establishment of a diagnosis
Alternative to community care if the person with bipolar disorder lacks adequate support in the community
Respite for the carer or carers

the psychiatric hospital to be a place of safety (or both). In some cases, attendance at a day hospital during office hours only may provide people with a more tolerable alternative to hospital admission.

A minority of people with a mood disorder who need to be admitted to a psychiatric hospital refuse to be admitted, usually because they lack insight into their mental illness. In many countries – and certainly in all industrialized countries – there are special legal provisions to protect such people from the consequences of their illness. In England and Wales, provisions for compulsory admission and treatment of mental illness are contained in the Mental Health Act 1983. The equivalent legislation in Scotland is the Mental Health (Care and Treatment) (Scotland) Act 2003, and in Northern Ireland it is the Mental Health (Northern Ireland) Order 1986. People admitted to hospital under one of these Acts do not lose all their rights to make decisions about their future. Soon after being admitted to hospital, the person has his or her rights explained by a member of staff, and the person can also ask for this information in writing.

The Mental Health Act

In England and Wales, the Mental Health Act is the principal Act governing not only the compulsory admission and detention of people to a psychiatric hospital, but also their treatment, discharge from hospital and aftercare. People with a mental disorder as defined by the Act can be detained under the Act in the interests of their health or safety or in the interests of the safety of others. To minimize the potential for abuse, the Act specifically excludes as mental disorder promiscuity, other 'immoral' conduct, sexual deviancy, and dependence on alcohol or drugs. Note that Scotland is governed by the Mental Health (Care and Treatment) (Scotland) Act 2003 and Northern Ireland by the Mental Health (Northern Ireland) Order 1986.

What is a 'section 2'?

Two of the most common 'sections' of the Mental Health Act that are used to admit people with a mental disorder to a psychiatric hospital are the so-called sections 2 and 3. Section 2 allows for an admission for assessment and treatment that can last for up to 28 days. An application for a section 2 is usually made by an Approved Mental Health Professional (AMHP) with special training in mental health and must be recommended by two doctors, one of whom must have special experience in the diagnosis and treatment of mental disorders. Under a section 2, treatment can be given, but only if this treatment is aimed at treating the mental disorder or conditions directly resulting from the mental disorder (so, for example, treatment for an inflamed appendix cannot be given under the Act, although treatment for deliberate self-harm might). A section 2 can be 'discharged' or revoked at any time by the Responsible Clinician (usually the consultant psychiatrist in charge), by the hospital managers, or by the nearest relative. Furthermore, a person under a section 2 can appeal against the section, in which case his or her appeal is heard by a specially constituted tribunal. The claimant is represented by a solicitor who helps him or her make a case in favour of discharge to the tribunal. The tribunal is by nature adversarial, and it falls upon members of the detained person's care team to argue the case for continued detention. This can be quite trying for both the claimant and his or her care team, and it can at times undermine the claimant's trust in the care team.

What is a 'section 3'?

A person can be detained under a 'section 3' after a conclusive period of assessment under a section 2. Alternatively, he or she can be detained directly under a section 3 if his or her diagnosis has already been established by the care team and is not in reasonable doubt. Section 3 corresponds to an admission for treatment and lasts for up to six months. As for a section 2, it is usually applied for by an AMHP with special training in mental health and approved by two doctors, one of whom must have special experience in the diagnosis and treatment of mental disorders. Treatment can only be given under a section 3 if it is aimed at treating the mental disorder or conditions directly resulting from the mental disorder. After the first three months, any treatment requires either the consent of the person being treated or the recommendation of a second doctor. A section 3 can be discharged at any time by the Responsible Clinician (usually the consultant psychiatrist in charge), by the hospital managers, or by the nearest relative. Furthermore, the person under a section 3 can appeal against the section, in which case his or her appeal is heard by a specially constituted tribunal, as explained above. If the person still needs to be detained after six months, the section 3 can be renewed for further periods.

What is 'aftercare'?

If a person has been detained under section 3 of the Mental Health Act, he or she is automatically placed under a 'section 117' at the time of his or her discharge from section 3. Section 117 corresponds to 'aftercare' and places a duty on the local health authority and local social services authority to provide the person with a care package aimed at rehabilitation and relapse prevention. Although the person is under no obligation to accept aftercare, in some cases he or she may also be placed under a 'Supervised Community Treatment' or Guardianship to ensure that he or she receives aftercare. Under Supervised Community Treatment, the person is made subject to certain conditions; if these conditions are not met, he or she can be recalled into hospital.

What other Sections of the Mental Health Act are commonly used?

Commonly used sections of the Mental Health Act are summarized in Table 6.5 on pages 54–5.

Reform of the Mental Health Act

In July 1998, the Government announced its intention to reform the Mental Health Act 1983, and this culminated nine years later in the Mental Health Act 2007, which amends the Mental Health Act 1983. The Mental Health Act 2007 introduced a number of significant changes, some of the most important being:

- A single definition of mental disorder
- The introduction of a requirement that a person cannot be detained for treatment unless appropriate treatment is available (the 'appropriate medical treatment test'), rather than the previous situation in which a person could not be detained unless he or she could be treated (the 'treatability test')
- A broadening of the range of professionals who can take on the functions which were performed by the Approved Social Worker (ASW, to be renamed 'Approved Mental Heath Professional') and the Responsible Medical Officer (RMO, to be renamed 'Responsible Clinician').

Table 6.5 Commonly used sections of the Mental Health Act

Section	Description	Duration	Treatment	Application or recommendations	Discharge or renewal
2	Admission for assessment	28 days	Can be given, but note that the MHA only authorizes treatment of the mental disorder itself or conditions directly resulting from the mental disorder	Application by AMHP or nearest relative. Recommendation by two doctors (at least one must be Section 12-approved)	Person may appeal to tribunal. Can be discharged by RC, hospital managers or nearest relative. Usually converted to Section 3 if a longer period of detention is required
3	Admission for treatment	6 months	Can be given for first 3 months, then consent or second opinion is needed.	Application by AMHP or nearest relative. Recommendation by two doctors (at least one must be Section 12-approved).	Person may appeal to tribunal. Can be discharged by RC, hospital managers or nearest relative. Can be renewed if needed.

AC, Approved Clinician; AMHP, Approved Mental Health Professional; MHA, Mental Health Act; RC, Responsible Clinician; Section 12-approved, Section 12 approval is usually granted to psychiatrists having obtained Membership of the Royal College of Psychiatrists (MRCPsych) or having more than 3 years' experience.

Table 6.5   contd

Section	Description	Duration	Treatment	Application or recommendations	Discharge or renewal
4	Emergency admission for assessment (used in lieu of a Section 2)	72 hours	Consent needed unless treatment is being given under common law	Application by AMHP or nearest relative. Recommendation by any doctor	Person cannot appeal. Can be discharged by RC only
5(2)	Emergency holding order (person already admitted to hospital on an informal basis)	72 hours	Consent needed unless treatment is being given under common law	Recommendation from the doctor or AC in charge of the patient's care of their nominated deputy	Person cannot appeal. Can be discharged by RC only
5(4)	Emergency holding order (person already admitted to hospital on an informal basis)	6 hours	Consent needed unless treatment is being given under common law	Recommendation from a registered mental nurse	Person cannot appeal
117	Automatically applies if a person has been detained under Section 3. Under Section 117 it is the duty of the local health authority and the local social services authority to provide after-care. Unlike under Supervised Community Treatment, there is no obligation for the person to accept it.				

- The ability for a person to make an application to displace (or change) his or her nearest relative, and the ability for civil partners to be the nearest relative
- The replacement of supervised discharge with 'Supervised Community Treatment', with a power to recall a person into hospital if he or she does not comply with certain conditions
- Statutory advocacy for detained patients
- New safeguards for electroconvulsive therapy

The Care Programme Approach

The longer-term care and treatment of people accepted into specialist mental health-care services is usually planned at one or several Care Programme Approach (CPA) meetings attended by both the person with bipolar disorder and his or her carers. These meetings are useful for establishing the context of the person's illness; evaluating his or her current personal circumstances; assessing his or her medical, psychological and social needs; and formulating a detailed care and treatment plan to ensure that these needs are met. As well as ensuring that the bipolar sufferer takes his or her medication and is regularly seen by a psychiatrist or CPN, this care and treatment plan may involve a number of psychological or social interventions such as attendance at self-help groups, carer education and support, home help, and cognitive behavioural therapy. A care co-ordinator, most often a CPN or social worker, is appointed to ensure that the care and treatment plan is implemented and revised in light of changing needs and circumstances. The people who generally attend CPA meetings are listed in Table 6.6.

At the outcome of a CPA meeting the bipolar sufferer should feel that his or her needs and circumstances have been understood, and that the care plan that he or she has helped to formulate closely reflects these.

Table 6.6   People who regularly attend Care Programme Approach meetings

The person with bipolar disorder

Relatives or advocates of the person with bipolar disorder

The Responsible Clinician (usually a consultant psychiatrist)

Other psychiatrists

The GP

The care co-ordinator (most often a community psychiatric nurse or social worker)

A community psychiatric nurse

A social worker

An occupational therapist

7

Treatment I: Antipsychotic medication

Introduction

The choice of medication in bipolar disorder is largely determined by the current symptoms. In a manic episode the treatment most often used is antipsychotic medication. In a depressive episode, the treatment most often used is antidepressant medication, often in conjunction with a mood stabilizer to avoid manic switch (that is, over-treatment into mania). In rare instances, a depressive episode may be so severe or unresponsive that electroconvulsive therapy is indicated. Even more rarely, electroconvulsive therapy might also be used for mania that cannot be treated by medication, either because it is unresponsive to medication or because medication is contraindicated. Finally, in the longer term the patient should be on a mood stabilizer to prevent further relapses into mania and depression. In addition, there are a number of psychological and social interventions that can play a major role not only in improving outcome, but also in improving quality of life.

Antipsychotic medication

Is antipsychotic medication always needed in the treatment of mania?

People with mania are usually at high risk of harming themselves or others, and for this reason mania is considered to be a medical emergency. Although psychological and social treatments have an important role to play in the management of bipolar disorder, medication is always needed for the treatment of mania. If a person with mania is not already on a long-term mood stabilizer, the most common practice is to start an antipsychotic medication and to wait for the person with bipolar disorder to get better before a long-term mood stabilizer is started. Often, people with mania are already on a long-term mood stabilizer such as lithium or valproate, in which case it is common to continue the mood stabilizer and add an antipsychotic medication.

Antipsychotic medication is fast-acting and effective, but relatively high doses are required and, unlike a mood stabilizer, antipsychotic medication does not protect against future depressive episodes. For these reasons it is sometimes preferable to start a mood stabilizer instead of an antipsychotic medication, or to start both at the same time. The disadvantage of starting a mood stabilizer during a manic episode is that the person with bipolar disorder often cannot participate in the decision to start the mood stabilizer, and this compromises his or her chances of taking the mood stabilizer in the long term. Once started, antipsychotic medication should be continued until full remission has been achieved. In some cases, antipsychotic medication may be continued as a long-term treatment, particularly if the bipolar disorder is characterized by prominent psychotic symptoms, mixed states, rapid cycling, or treatment resistance.

In the initial stages of treatment the bipolar sufferer may be highly agitated and difficult to manage, and a very fast-acting sedative such as lorazepam may be given in addition to an antipsychotic or mood stabilizer. If the person with bipolar disorder is sleep-deprived, a sleeping tablet such as temazepam or zopiclone may also be given. In contrast, any antidepressant medication should be tapered off and stopped.

Many people understandably do not like taking too much medication because they are frightened of becoming addicted to pills or of suffering from undesirable side effects. Like all medication, antipsychotic medication can have side effects, but it is not in any sense addictive. Adequate management of the situation involves balancing the risks and benefits of treatment with antipsychotic medication and reassessing that balance in the light of changing circumstances. It is important to remember that not all people taking antipsychotic medication suffer from side effects, and that for many of those who do, the side effects are only mild or temporary. See below for an explanation of the side effects of antipsychotic medication.

How does antipsychotic medication work?

You may recall from chapter 2 that the symptoms of mania result from an excess of certain excitatory neurotransmitters, or chemical messengers, in the brain. These neurotransmitters include the monoamines dopamine, noradrenaline, and serotonin. Antipsychotics are effective in the treatment of mania principally because they block the effects of dopamine in certain parts of the brain.

Which antipsychotic medication is the best one for me?

Current treatment guidelines for the treatment of mania recommend starting with one of the more recent (so-called atypical) antipsychotics, which are less likely to produce certain types of disturbing side effects called extrapyramidal side effects (see below) than the older (so called typical) antipsychotics. There are several atypical antipsychotics; quetiapine, olanzapine, and risperidone are the most commonly prescribed ones. While these antipsychotics are, on balance, similarly effective, each has a slightly different side-effect profile, which the person with bipolar disorder, aided by his or her doctor and carers, can choose from. In addition, some antipsychotics come in different forms, which can make taking them easier. For example, they may come in liquid form or as an oral dispersible tablet (ODT) that dissolves in the mouth. The various factors involved in choosing an antipsychotic medication are listed in Table 7.1.

Table 7.1   **Principal factors involved in choosing an antipsychotic medication**

Initially

Particular side effect(s) that the person with bipolar disorder is keen to avoid

Any previous side effects that he or she found to be unacceptable

Difficulties that he or she anticipates in taking the antipsychotic medication in standard tablet form

Later in the course of treatment

Effectiveness of antipsychotic in controlling the symptoms

Current side effects that the person with bipolar disorder finds to be unacceptable

Difficulties that he or she has in taking the antipsychotic in standard tablet form

What are the side effects of antipsychotic medication?

Antipsychotics are effective in the treatment of mania principally because they block the effects of dopamine in the brain. Unfortunately, by doing this, they also cause a number of side effects (see Figure 7.1). If an antipsychotic blocks the effects of dopamine in a part of the brain called the nigrostriatal tract, this can lead to extrapyramidal side effects, which involve a disturbance of muscle function. The four recognized types of extrapyramidal side effects are explained in Table 7.2 on page 63. If an antipsychotic blocks the effects of dopamine in a part of the brain called the tuberoinfundibular tract, this can lead to an increase in the hormone prolactin (hyperprolactinaemia), which can cause loss of libido and, in men, erectile dysfunction.

Antipsychotic medication can also interfere with other neurotransmitters in the brain, and this may potentially result in further side effects. An important and common side effect is sedation, although some degree of sedation is beneficial in people with manic symptoms. Another important and common side effect is weight gain, which can place the person with bipolar disorder at a long-term risk of heart disease and

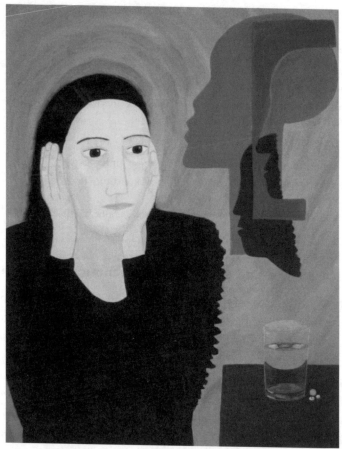

Figure 7.1 'Medication', a painting by Philippa King. The artist explains, 'The side effects I was experiencing on antipsychotic medication were tremors in my arms and hands (illustrated by the wavy line of the sleeve), a dry mouth (another reason for including a glass of water in the picture), and weight gain.'

diabetes. For these reasons it is important to have your physical health monitored, to avoid smoking, to develop and maintain healthy eating habits, and to take regular exercise. It is especially important that you heed this advice if you are on long-term antipsychotic medication or if you frequently require

Table 7.2 Extrapyramidal side effects of antipsychotics

Acute dystonias	Acute dystonias involve painful contractions of a muscle or muscle group, most commonly in the neck, eyes, and trunk. They are usually easily recognized and successfully treated with anticholinergic medication such as procyclidine, orphenadrine, or benzhexol
Akathisia	Akathisia involves a distressing feeling of inner restlessness, manifested by fidgety leg movements, shuffling of the feet, and pacing. As akathisia is readily confused with the symptoms of mania, it can sometimes be difficult to recognize. Treatment usually involves reducing the dose of antipsychotic or changing to another antipsychotic
Parkinson-like symptoms	Parkinson-like symptoms principally involve three features: tremor, muscular rigidity, and difficulty starting movements. Parkinson-like symptoms may respond to anticholinergic medication, although it is often preferable to reduce the dose of antipsychotic or change to another antipsychotic
Tardive dyskinesia	Tardive dyskinesia usually occurs after several months or years of antipsychotic treatment and is often irreversible. It involves involuntary, repetitive, purposeless movements of the tongue, lips, face, trunk, and extremities. The movements may be generalized or affect only certain muscle groups, typically the muscles around the mouth. There is no consistently beneficial treatment, and the condition may be exacerbated by anticholinergic medication. Since the advent of atypical antipsychotics, tardive dyskinesia has become considerably less common

treatment with antipsychotic medication. Other common side effects of antipsychotic medication include orthostatic hypotension (dizziness upon sitting up and standing) and so-called anticholinergic side effects such as dry mouth, blurred vision, and constipation.

Any side effects that have not been mentioned above are comparatively uncommon, and they may vary from one antipsychotic medication to another.

Table 7.3   Comparison of the side-effect profiles of four atypical antipsychotics

	Extrapyramidal side effects	Hyperprolactinaemia	Sedation	Weight gain	Orthostatic hypotension	Anticholinergic side effects
Risperidone	+	++	+	+	++	0/+
Olanzapine	0/+	+	++	+++	+	+/++
Quetipaine	0/+	0/+	++	++	++	0/+
Clozapine	0	0	+++	+++	+++	+++

As there are a number of antipsychotic medications to choose from, you need not expect to suffer from side effects that you find unacceptable. If you feel that you are suffering from such side effects then speak to your psychiatrist or CPN about it. Many side effects of antipsychotic medication can be controlled by diet and lifestyle changes, or by other medications that can be prescribed for you. Alternatively, the dose of the antipsychotic medication can be reduced or the antipsychotic medication can be changed to a different one.

The side effects most commonly seen in four atypical antipsychotic medications are summarised in Table 7.3.

What is neuroleptic malignant syndrome?

Neuroleptic malignant syndrome (NMS) is a rare but potentially dangerous reaction to antipsychotic medication. Symptoms include tiredness, confusion, dizziness, palpitations, muscle rigidity, and fever. NMS can sometimes be mistaken for other conditions such as an infection or the serotonin syndrome (see page 72). The mainstay of treatment involves stopping the antipsychotic medication and admitting the person to hospital for monitoring and support.

Aripiprazole

Aripiprazole is a relatively novel, so-called third-generation anti-psychotic medication that has been described as a 'dopamine-serotonin system stabilizer'. It has been demonstrated to have good efficacy in treating manic symptoms and to be better tolerated than other atypical antipsychotic medication. Principal side effects include headache, anxiety, insomnia, nausea, vomiting, and light-headedness but *not* extrapyramidal side effects, hyper-prolactinaemia, sedation, or weight gain. As our understanding of bipolar disorder improves, novel treatments such as aripiprazole are likely to continue emerging.

Can I take antipsychotic medication if I am pregnant or breast-feeding?

There are some scientific data to suggest that exposure to anti-psychotic medication during the first trimester of pregnancy is linked to a small additional risk of congenital abnormalities in the foetus. However, withholding antipsychotic medication may result in behavioural disturbances that expose the mother and foetus to much higher levels of overall risk. For this reason, pregnant women are generally advised to remain on antipsychotic medication.

Antipsychotic medication is excreted into breast milk, but except in the case of clozapine, breast-fed infants do not seem to suffer from this. Thus, a mother may decide to breast-feed while remaining on antipsychotic medication.

What should I ask my doctor before I start on antipsychotic medication?

Questions that you or your carer might want to ask your doctor before you start taking antipsychotic medication include:

- How will it help me?
- How should I take it?
- How long will it take to work?
- What side effects am I risking, and is there anything I can do to avoid or reduce them?
- Whom should I speak to if there is a problem? How can I get hold of him or her?
- How long do I need to take the antipsychotic medication for?

How is antipsychotic medication started?

If a person with bipolar disorder is starting on an antipsychotic medication for the first time, the starting dose is normally relatively small so as to minimize any potential side effects. The dose is then increased according to the response, up to the minimum dose that is effective for him or her (this dose varies according to a large number of factors, such as the severity of the manic episode, age, sex, and weight).

What if I find taking antipsychotic medication difficult?

Some people may be reluctant to take their medication because, owing to the nature of their illness, they do not realize or accept that they are ill. Other reasons for not taking medication include side effects, delusional beliefs about the medication (for example, that it is poison), fear of becoming addicted to the medication, poor concentration or motivation, and a poor relationship with the doctor or a key worker.

Missing tablets can lead to a relapse or recurrence of symptoms, so it is particularly important for both you and your family to discuss any difficulties in taking your medication and to have these difficulties addressed as far as is possible. For example, your psychiatrist may be able to reduce the dose of your antipsychotic medication, change your antipsychotic medication to a different one, or simplify your medication schedule.

What if my antipsychotic medication does not work?

If your symptoms do not respond to the chosen atypical antipsychotic after an adequate trial period, the dose can be increased. If your symptoms still do not respond, the antipsychotic can be stopped and another one started. Alternatively, a mood stabilizer such as valproate can be started or added (see Chapter 8). If your symptoms continue to resist treatment, an atypical antipsychotic called clozapine can be considered. Although clozapine is the most effective antipsychotic available, it requires registration with a monitoring service and, in the initial period, daily monitoring of vital signs as well as weekly blood tests. The blood tests monitor the white blood cell count, which can drop dangerously in up to 1 per cent of people on clozapine. White blood cells fight off infections, so a drop in the white cell count can suddenly leave the body exposed to danger.

How long should I take my antipsychotic medication for?

Once started, antipsychotic medication should be continued until full remission of manic symptoms has been achieved. In some cases, antipsychotic medication may be continued as a long-term treatment (often with a mood stabilizer), particularly if the bipolar disorder is characterized by prominent psychotic symptoms, mixed states, rapid cycling, or treatment resistance. The antipsychotic medication most commonly used for long-term treatment is olanzapine.

Table 7.4   Principal advantages and disadvantages of oral versus depot antipsychotic medication

	Advantages	*Disadvantages*
Oral medication	Short duration of action Flexible	Variable absorption from the gut Potential for poor compliance Potential for misuse and overdose
Depot medication	Less potential for poor compliance Less potential for abuse and overdose Regular contact with community psychiatric nurse or practice nurse who gives the injection	Needle injections Potential delayed side effects Potential prolonged side effects Potential damage to relationship between the person with bipolar disorder and his or her carers

What is 'depot' antipsychotic medication?

Some people who have difficulties taking their antipsychotic medication may benefit from receiving it in the form of an injectable long-term preparation or 'depot', instead of the usual oral tablet or oral liquid form. The principal advantages and disadvantages of depot versus oral antipsychotic medication are listed in Table 7.4. Before starting a person on a depot, it is usual to administer an oral test dose first. After about 7 days, the first depot dose is administered, and the dose is then increased at regular intervals as the oral antipsychotic is decreased and stopped. Depot injections are usually given every 7 or 14 days.

Commonly used antipsychotic medications

The commonly used typical, atypical, and depot antipsychotic medications are listed in Table 7.5.

Table 7.5 Commonly used atypical, typical, and depot antipsychotic medications

Antipsychotic medication	Trade name	Licensed daily dose range in adults under the age of 65
Atypical antipsychotics (introduced from 1990)		
Olanzapine	Zyprexa	15–20mg
Quetiapine	Seroquel	100–800mg (usual dose range 400–800mg)
Clozapine	Clozaril, Denzapine	25–900mg (usual dose range 200–450mg)
Risperidone	Risperdal	2–16mg (rarely exceeds 10mg)
Amisulpiride	Solian	400–1200mg
Aripiprazole	Abilify	10–30mg
Typical antipsychotics (introduced from 1950s)		
Chlorpromazine	Largactil	75–1000mg
Fluphenazine	Modecate/Moditen	2–20mg
Haloperidol	Haldol/Dozic/Serenace	3–30mg
Pimozide	Orap	2–20mg
Flupenthixol	Depixol	3–18mg
Zuclopenthixol	Clopixol	20–150mg
Sulpiride	Dolmatil/Sulpitil/Sulpor	400–2400mg
Depot antipsychotics		
Risperidone	Risperdal Consta	Maximum dose: 50mg every 2 weeks
Fluphenazine decanoate	Modecate	Test dose: 12.5mg; maximum dose: 100mg every 2 weeks
Flupenthixol decanoate	Depixol	Test dose: 20mg; maximum dose: 400mg per week
Zuclopenthixol decanoate	Clopixol	Test dose: 100mg; maximum dose: 600mg per week
Pipiotazine palmitate	Piportil depot	Test dose: 25mg; maximum: 200mg every 4 weeks

Note that many of these antipsychotic medications (particularly the typical and depot ones) are not specifically licensed for the treatment of mania, but are sometimes used nonetheless.

8

II: Antidepressant medication and electroconvulsive therapy

Antidepressant medication

What is the role of antidepressant medication in bipolar disorder?

In bipolar disorder the most commonly used treatment for a depressive episode is antidepressant medication, often in conjunction with a mood stabilizer or antipsychotic medication to avoid manic switch (that is, over-treatment into mania). All antidepressants can result in manic switch, so in most cases an antidepressant should be avoided if depressive symptoms are only mild, and the antidepressant, if used, should be tapered off and stopped once depressive symptoms have resolved. In rare instances, a bipolar depression may be so severe or unresponsive that electroconvulsive therapy is indicated. Other medications that are sometimes advocated for the treatment of bipolar depression are lithium, valproate, lamotrigine, carbamazepine, and antipsychotic medication (see also Chapter 9).

What types of antidepressants are there?

Antidepressants are often chosen according to local practice or guidelines or according to the personal choice of the person with bipolar disorder. In the treatment of bipolar depression, no one antidepressant appears to be significantly more effective than any other, although one antidepressant can be effective in one person but not in another. Each antidepressant and antidepressant type has a slightly different side-effect profile, and this can be an important factor in choosing one over another.

Table 8.1 Commonly used selective serotonin reuptake inhibitors in the treatment of bipolar depression

Antidepressant	Trade name	Licensed daily dose range in adults under the age of 65, and form
Citalopram	Cipramil	20–60mg, tablets or oral drops
Escitalopram	Cipralex	10–20mg, tablets
Fluoxetine	Prozac	20–60mg, tablets or liquid
Fluvoxamine	Faverin	50–300mg, tablets
Paroxetine	Seroxat	20–50mg, tablets or liquid
Sertraline	Lustral	50–200mg, tablets

There are several different types of antidepressants, but the most commonly prescribed antidepressants belong to the class of serotonin-selective reuptake inhibitors (SSRIs) (see Table 8.1). SSRIs, such as fluoxetine, paroxetine, sertraline, and citalopram, prevent the reuptake (or 'mopping up') of the chemical messenger serotonin in the brain. Other antidepressant types prescribed include noradrenaline reuptake inhibitors (NARIs) and serotonin and noradrenaline reuptake inhibitors (SNRIs), but these tend to be used as second-line treatment (that is, if treatment with an SSRI fails). The older tricyclic antidepressants increase the risk of manic switch; for this reason, they are usually avoided in the treatment of bipolar depression.

How should I take my antidepressant medication?

If you have been prescribed an SSRI, you should be aware that they can take 10–20 days to start having an effect. During this period, they may cause mild yet bothersome side effects, but these tend to resolve during the first month of treatment. Thus, it is important to continue taking your antidepressant medication, even though it may initially seem like it is doing more harm than good. SSRIs are normally taken once a day, every morning. If you fail to respond to your antidepressant medication despite taking it for an adequate length of time, your doctor can increase its dose or try another antidepressant medication from the same class or from a different class. If this also fails and symptoms of depression remain severe, electroconvulsive therapy (ECT) can be considered (see below).

What are the side effects of SSRIs?

SSRIs, like all medication, can have side effects, but they are generally less dangerous and better tolerated than those of older types of antidepressants. As their side effects are comparatively mild, SSRIs are particularly useful in the elderly and the physically ill. Side effects include dry mouth, nausea, vomiting, diarrhoea, dizziness, sedation, sexual dysfunction, agitation, akathisia (see page 63) and, very rarely, parkinsonism (see page 63), and convulsions. Some SSRIs, such as fluoxetine, fluvoxamine, and paroxetine inhibit certain enzymes in the liver and so interfere with the metabolism of some other medications. If you are on any other medications, speak to your doctor about these.

What is the SSRI discontinuation syndrome?

The SSRI discontinuation syndrome consists of headache, dizziness, shock-like sensations, paraesthesia, gastrointestinal symptoms, lethargy, insomnia, and change in mood (depression, anxiety, agitation). It occurs most frequently after the abrupt discontinuation of paroxetine.

Some people fear that SSRIs may be addictive because they have heard or read about the SSRI discontinuation syndrome. However, SSRIs are not addictive in the sense that people do not experience a 'high' from them, and do not seek or crave them in the way that they might a drug of abuse such as cocaine or heroin.

What is the serotonin syndrome?

The serotonin syndrome is a rare but potentially dangerous syndrome resulting from increased serotonin activity in the brain. It is typically caused by SSRIs but can be caused by other medications too, such as tricyclic antidepressants and lithium. Symptoms include:

- Psychological symptoms – agitation, confusion
- Neurological symptoms – tremor, muscle jerks, seizures
- Other symptoms – fever, palpitations, dizziness

If a person is both on antipsychotic medication and an SSRI, serotonin syndrome can be difficult to tell apart from NMS (see page 64). Management of the serotonin syndrome involves stopping the SSRI and admitting the person to hospital for monitoring and physical support.

What are the side effects of some of the other types of antidepressant?

Reboxetine, a NARI, is less likely than the SSRIs to result in manic switch. More common side effects are dry mouth, constipation, and insomnia. SNRIs such as venlafaxine have a similar side-effect profile to that of the SSRIs and may cause hypertension and heart disease. Compared with other antidepressants, the noradrenaline- and serotonin-specific antidepressant (NaSSa) mirtazepine tends to increase appetite and result in less sexual dysfunction. Common side effects of mirtazepine include weight gain, sedation, and dry mouth.

Electroconvulsive therapy

What is the role of electroconvulsive therapy in bipolar disorder?

Electroconvulsive therapy (ECT) has been demonstrated to be safe and effective in the treatment of mood symptoms that are both severe and unresponsive to medication. In the context of bipolar disorder, electroconvulsive therapy may be used either in the treatment of severe and unresponsive depression or, even less commonly, in the treatment of severe and unresponsive mania. It can be particularly useful in the presence of marked psychotic symptoms, retardation (or slowing down) of movement, or high suicidal risk. The Mental Health Act 2007 (see Chapter 6) introduces new safeguards for the use of ECT. In summary, ECT may not be given to a person with the capacity to refuse to consent to it, and it may only be given to a person without the capacity to refuse consent to it if this does not conflict with any advance directive, decision of a donee or deputy, or decision of the Court of Protection.

What does modern ECT look like?

In pre-modern times it was observed that convulsions induced by camphor could improve psychotic illnesses such as schizophrenia and depression. In 1933, the German psychiatrist Sakel began the practice of using insulin injections to induce convulsions, but a period of panic and impending doom prior to the convulsion made the treatment very difficult to tolerate. The Hungarian psychiatrist Meduna replaced insulin with metrazol, but similar problems remained. Then in 1938 the Italian neuropsychiatrist Cerletti began the practice of applying electric current directly to the scalp. Cerletti's method soon superseded Sakel's insulin injections and Meduna's metrazol injections as the least unpopular method of inducing convulsions. The advent of suitable short-acting anaesthetics and muscle relaxants in the 1950s made the procedure much safer by reducing complications such as muscle pains and broken teeth. Today, the patient is asleep and the convulsions are so small that in most cases they can barely be seen.

Can ECT be used in all people?

The short reply is yes. ECT is a potentially life-saving treatment, and the benefits and the risks need to be weighed up in each case. Thus, while there are no absolute contraindications for ECT, relative contraindications include:

- Cardiovascular disease
- Dementing illnesses
- Epilepsy and other neurological disorders
- Raised intracranial pressure, for example, as a result of head injury or a brain tumour
- Cervical spine disease

Note that pregnancy and old age are *not* contraindications to ECT, and that ECT is sometimes preferred to drug therapy during pregnancy.

How is ECT delivered?

The patient is given a standard anaesthetic such as propofol and a muscle relaxant such as suxamethonium. Once the patient is asleep, the modern approach is to deliver constant-current, brief-pulse ECT at a voltage that is above the patient's seizure threshold. In many cases, the seizure is barely visible and so must be monitored using an electroencephalograph (EEG) recording. The choice of bilateral (two-sided) or right-sided unilateral ECT should be made on a case-by-case basis, although many centres practice only bilateral ECT. Bilateral ECT is more effective than unilateral ECT, but unilateral ECT has fewer cognitive side effects (see below). Most patients respond to a course of four to eight ECT treatments, usually delivered over a period of two to four weeks. Prior to starting a course of ECT treatments, a patient should have a physical examination, an electrocardiograph (ECG), and some blood tests and should not eat or drink (unless as instructed – for instance, to take medication) from the previous midnight. Informed consent is needed except if being treated under the provision of the Mental Health Act.

What are the side effects of ECT?

The side effects of ECT are generally mild and include:

- The side effects of the anaesthetic

- Headache
- Muscle aches
- Nausea
- Temporary confusion
- Temporary memory impairment

Mortality is similar to that of general anaesthesia in minor surgical procedures and mostly results from cardiovascular complications such as arrhythmias. Although memory impairment is a recognized side effect, most patients receiving ECT actually feel their memory improving as their depression lifts or their concentration improves. Interestingly, emerging evidence suggests that the use of repetitive transcranial magnetic stimulation (rTMS) may in some cases provide an alternative to ECT in depression and other psychiatric disorders.

9

III: Mood stabilizers

Lithium

Of all our conversations, I remember most vividly [Robert Lowell's] words about the new drug, lithium carbonate, which had such good results and gave him reason to believe he was cured: 'It's terrible, Bob, to think that all I've suffered, and all the suffering I've caused, might have arisen from the lack of a little salt in my brain'.

Robert Giroux

I have often asked myself whether, given the choice, I would choose to have manic–depressive illness. If lithium were not available to me, or didn't work for me, the answer would be a simple no and it would be an answer laced with terror. But lithium does work for me, and therefore I suppose I can afford to pose the question. Strangely enough I think I would choose to have it. It's complicated.

Kay Redfield Jamison, *An Unquiet Mind*

The Australian psychiatrist and researcher John Cade serendipitously discovered the calming properties of lithium in 1948, and the naturally occurring ion became the first effective treatment for bipolar disorder. Today lithium is commonly used in the long-term treatment of bipolar disorder to prevent further relapses of both mania and depression, and sometimes also in the short-term treatment of manic and hypomanic episodes. In the long-term treatment of bipolar disorder, it decreases the relapse rates by about one-third, but is more effective against mania than against depression. It is also the only mood stabilizer that has been scientifically proven to decrease the risk of suicide. Despite its popularity, its mode of action is still unclear.

It is understood to have a range of effects in the brain, including effects on certain chemical messengers and their receptors.

Ideally, lithium should be started only if there is a clear intention to continue it for at least three years, since poor compliance and intermittent treatment may precipitate episodes of 'rebound' mania or hypomania. The starting dose of lithium is normally cautious, but depends on the type of preparation used – for example, lithium carbonate versus lithium citrate. A blood test to determine the serum level of lithium needs to be taken about 12 hours after the first dose. Further such blood tests then need to be taken at 5–7 day intervals until the serum level of lithium is stable, and thereafter at three- or four-monthly intervals. These blood tests need to be taken because serum lithium levels need to be within a relatively narrow range, or 'therapeutic window', of about 0.5–1.0 millimoles per litre (or 0.8–1.0 millimoles per litre in the short-term treatment of manic and hypomanic episodes). If the serum level of lithium is less than about 0.5 millimoles per litre, beneficial effects are limited; if it is more than about 1.0 millimoles per litre, side effects and toxic effects are more likely.

The toxic effects of lithium are usually experienced if serum levels exceed 1.5 millimoles per litre. They include anorexia, nausea, vomiting, diarrhoea, coarse tremor, difficulty articulating speech, clumsiness, unsteadiness, and, in severe cases, fits and loss of consciousness. Lithium is cleared out of the body through the kidneys, and serum levels of lithium depend on kidney function. For this reason, it is important to check kidney function before lithium is started. This is usually achieved by carrying out a simple blood test.

The side effects of lithium can occur even when serum lithium levels are within the therapeutic window, and can be divided into short-term and long-term side effects (see Table 9.1). Short-term side effects include a stuffy nose and a metallic taste in the mouth, fine tremor, nausea, diarrhoea, muscle weakness, thirst,

Table 9.1   Side effects of lithium

Short-term	Long-term
Stuffy nose	Swelling ('oedema')
Metallic taste in the mouth	Weight gain
Fine tremor	Skin: exacerbation of acne and psoriasis
Nausea	Thyroid: goitre and hypothyroidism
Diarrhoea	Kidneys: renal damage, diabetes insipidus
Muscle weakness	Heart: cardiotoxicity
Passing a lot of urine ('polyuria')	
Drinking a lot of water ('polydipsia')	

Before lithium is started, it is standard practice to take simple blood test to check kidney and thyroid function, and to record a tracing of the heart.

and passing a lot of urine. In the long term, lithium can cause swelling and weight gain and make certain skin conditions such as acne and psoriasis flare up. Because lithium can affect the thyroid gland and the kidneys, simple blood tests need to be taken at six-monthly intervals to monitor thyroid and kidney function. Lithium can also affect the conduction of electrical impulses in the heart, and for this reason it is standard practice to record a tracing of the heart (an ECG) before starting treatment. If you are pregnant and on lithium, there is a very small chance that lithium might cause a malformation of the heart in the foetus. That having been said, the risk of this happening is less than one in 1,000, and this risk needs to be counterbalanced against the much higher risk of relapse if lithium is stopped or the dose decreased. As lithium is passed into breast milk, breast-feeding should be avoided.

Lithium has a response rate of about 75 per cent, or three in four, in the treatment of short-term manic and hypomanic episodes, but it takes several days to produce an effect. If lithium is effective and side effects are absent, not troublesome, or tolerable, it should be continued in the long term. If not, it can be stopped abruptly. In contrast, after long-term treatment it should only be stopped gradually over the course of two to three months to minimize the risk of precipitating an episode of rebound mania or hypomania. People who are on lithium should drink plenty of fluids and avoid reducing their salt intake, because dehydration and salt depletion can in some cases precipitate lithium toxicity.

Valproate, lamotrigine, and carbamazepine

The use of anticonvulsants (principally valproate and, more recently, lamotrigine) in the long-term treatment of bipolar disorder is increasing. Their precise mode of action in preventing relapses of bipolar disorder is as yet unclear.

Valproate, in the form of semisodium valproate (Depakote), is used alone or as an adjunct to lithium or other medications in the long-term and short-term treatment of bipolar disorder, and in the USA it has become the most frequently prescribed mood stabilizer. Compared with lithium, it has similar efficacy but a quicker onset of action. It is also of particular value in rapid-cycling bipolar disorder. Although valproate can have a number of side effects it is often better tolerated than lithium, particularly if lithium levels need to be maintained above 0.8 millimoles per litre. Side effects of valproate include nausea, tremor, tiredness, weight gain, hair loss, blood cell problems, and liver toxicity. During pregnancy, valproate can significantly increase the risk of malformations in the foetus; for this reason it may be avoided in women of child-bearing age. It is important to check blood cell counts and liver function before valproate is started and to continue monitoring these at six- to twelve-monthly intervals. This is usually achieved by carrying out a simple blood test.

In contrast to lithium, lamotrigine is more effective against relapses of depression than it is against relapses of mania, and it can be used both as a short-term treatment for relapses of depression and for long-term mood stabilization. Compared with the other mood stabilizers discussed here, lamotrigine has fewer side effects and does not usually require long-term monitoring with blood tests. However, monitoring of serum levels of lamotrigine may be required if it is being taken in combination with either valproate or carbamazepine because both of these other drugs affect the metabolism (or breakdown) of lamotrigine. Common side effects include dizziness, clumsiness and unsteadiness, sedation, insomnia, and nausea and vomiting. Other side effects include irritation of the oesophagus (or food pipe), blurred vision, skin rash, and severe skin reactions.

Carbamazepine may be used as a second- or third-line treatment in the long-term treatment of bipolar disorder, and is thought to be of particular value in treatment-resistant cases and in rapid cycling. Side effects include nausea, headache, dizziness, tiredness, double vision, clumsiness and unsteadiness, skin rashes, electrolyte disturbances, blood cell problems, and liver toxicity. Blood tests need to be done regularly to monitor liver function, blood cell counts, and electrolytes. If used in pregnancy, carbamazepine can result in malformations of the foetus, but it is not excreted into breast milk and so can be used during breast-feeding. Because carbamazepine activates certain enzymes in the liver, it can speed up the metabolism (or breakdown) of a number of other drugs such as antipsychotics, lamotrigine, and the oral contraceptive pill. For this reason, if you are about to start on carbamazepine, you should tell your doctor about any other medications that you are already taking.

How should I choose which mood stabilizer to use?

Your choice of mood stabilizer should ideally depend on several factors, including:

- The type of symptoms that you have

- Your response to previous treatments, if any
- Your physical health – for instance, the presence of obesity, diabetes, or kidney disease
- Your degree of motivation and level of compliance with medication
- Your personal preference

What if my chosen mood stabilizer does not work for me?

If you have frequent relapses despite being on a mood stabilizer, you can either change to a different mood stabilizer or start taking a second mood stabilizer in addition to the first one (for example, start taking valproate in addition to lithium). Should you start on such combination therapy, symptoms, side effects, and serum levels should be very closely monitored. If you continue having frequent relapses on combination therapy, your psychiatrist may refer you for a second opinion from a clinician with particular expertise in the treatment of bipolar disorder.

10

IV: Psychological and social interventions

Introduction

The care of a person with bipolar disorder is usually planned at one or several CPA meetings. These meetings are useful for establishing the context of the illness, evaluating current personal circumstances, and formulating a detailed care plan to ensure that medical, psychological, and social needs are met. As well as ensuring that the person with bipolar disorder is receiving medication and is regularly reviewed by a member of the mental health-care team, the care plan may in due course involve a number of psychosocial measures, possibly including – among others – patient and family education, cognitive behavioural therapy, illness self-management, self-help groups, and social and vocational skills training.

Although under-utilized, psychosocial measures such as these can, alongside medication, play an important role in reducing symptoms, preventing relapse and re-hospitalization, and helping you to take control over your illness.

Managing stress and anxiety

Stress and anxiety can make you more vulnerable to a relapse in your illness. You might recall that stress can result from life events such as losing a loved one, going through a divorce, losing your job, or falling ill. But it can also result from seemingly smaller 'background' stressors such as constant deadlines, frustrations, and conflicts. The cumulative effect of these can be

Table 10.1   Some of the symptoms of stress

Emotional symptoms	Anxiety, fear, irritability, anger, resentment, loss of confidence, depression
Psychological symptoms	Difficulty concentrating or making decisions, confusion, repetitive or circular thoughts
Physical symptoms	Dry mouth, tremor, sweatiness, racing heartbeat, chest tightness and difficulty breathing, muscle tension, headache, dizziness
Behavioural symptoms	Nervous habits such as pacing or nail biting, drinking more coffee and alcohol, eating too much or too little, sleeping poorly, acting brashly or unreasonably, losing your temper, being inconsiderate to others, neglecting your responsibilities

far greater than any single life event. The amount of stress that a person can handle is largely related to his or her coping and thinking styles and level of social skills. People with positive coping and thinking styles and good social skills are better able to diffuse stressful situations – for example, by doing something about them, putting them in their correct context, or simply talking about them and 'sharing the pain'.

The first step in dealing with stress is to be able to recognize its warning signs. Study Table 10.1 and then write down on a piece of paper how you feel when you become stressed. Next make a list of situations in which you feel that way. For each situation on your list, think about one or more strategies for avoiding the situation or making it less stressful.

See Table 10.2 for some examples of situation-specific strategies for reducing stress. However, there are also more general strategies that you can use for reducing stress. One common and effective strategy, called deep breathing, involves regulating your breathing:

• Breathe in through your nose and hold the air in for several seconds

Table 10.2   A number of situation-specific strategies for reducing stress

Stressful situations	Possible strategies for reducing stress
Arguing with Liz	Talk to Liz about how I am feeling and try to resolve matters See her less often Avoid talking to her about certain things Walk away from an argument Use deep breathing
Receiving bills that I can't pay	Ask a relative to help me with my finances Speak to a social worker to see what help I can get Phone the bank and try to reach an agreement

- Then purse your lips and gradually let the air out, making sure that you let out as much as you can
- Continue doing this until you are feeling more relaxed

A second strategy, often used in conjunction with deep breathing, involves relaxation exercises:

- Lying on your back, tighten the muscles in your toes for 10 seconds and then relax them completely
- Do the same for your feet, ankles, and calves, gradually working your way up your body until you reach your head and neck

Other strategies that you can use for reducing stress include listening to classical music (for example, Bach or Chopin), taking a hot bath, reading a book or surfing the internet, calling up or meeting a friend, practising yoga or meditation, and playing sports.

Lifestyle changes can help to reduce stress as well as increase your ability to cope with stress. Some lifestyle changes that you should consider include:

- Simplifying your life, even if this means doing less or doing only one thing at a time
- Having a schedule and keeping to it
- Getting enough sleep
- Exercising regularly (for example, walking, swimming, yoga)
- Eating a balanced diet
- Avoiding excessive caffeine or alcohol
- Taking time out to do the things that you like doing
- Connecting with others and sharing your problems with them
- Changing your thinking style: having realistic expectations, reframing problems, expressing your feelings, maintaining a sense of humour

Such lifestyle changes are good not only for managing stress but also for your physical health and quality of life. Though individually small and simple, their cumulative effect can make a real difference to your chances of making a good recovery and avoiding a relapse.

If coping with stress continues to be a problem, consider asking a member of your mental health-care team whether you can be given relaxation training.

Coping with voices

Sometimes voices can in themselves be a significant source of stress and distress. Simple strategies to reduce or eliminate voices include:

- Finding a trusted person to talk to about the voices
- Focusing your attention on an activity such as reading, gardening, singing, or listening to your favourite music
- Keeping a diary of the voices to help you to identify and avoid situations in which they arise
- Talking back to the voices: challenge them and ask them to

go away; if you are out in public, you can avoid attracting attention by talking into a mobile phone
- Managing your anxiety and stress using the techniques offered in this book
- Taking your medication as prescribed
- Avoiding drugs and alcohol

Fighting off depression

While it is important that you continue to take your prescribed medication, psychological (or talking) treatments can also be effective in the treatment of depression. Types of talking treatments that may be appropriate for depression in bipolar disorder are listed in Table 10.3. The type of talking treatment that is chosen, if any, depends on your personal circumstances and preferences, but often also on the resources that are available in your local area.

Table 10.3   Psychological or talking treatments that can be used for depression in bipolar disorder

Psychological treatment	What it involves
Counselling	Identification and resolution of current life difficulties Explanation, reassurance, and support
Cognitive–behavioural therapy	Identification of thinking errors and associated behaviours that occur in depression Correction of these thinking errors and behaviours
Interpersonal psychotherapy	A systematic and standardized treatment approach to personal relationships and life problems that may be contributing to depression
Family therapy	Identification and resolution of negative aspects of family relationships that may be contributing to depression Family education and support

Cognitive behavioural therapy

From Figure 10.1 it can be seen that cognitive behavioural therapy is a type of exploratory psychotherapy that is based on learning and cognitive theories. Developed by Aaron Beck in the 1960s, cognitive behavioural therapy is an increasingly common form of treatment for many psychiatric disorders. It is generally unsuitable during a manic episode, but it can help to combat depression, improve functional and social skills, and reduce the risk of future relapses. It is most often carried out on a one-to-one basis, but it can also sometimes be offered in small groups. In either case, it involves a limited number of sessions (typically between 10 and 20), each about 1 hour long. However, most of the work takes place outside the sessions (in the form of 'homework'). The person with bipolar disorder and a trained therapist (who may be a psychologist, a counsellor, a doctor, or a nurse) develop a shared understanding of the person's current problems and try to understand them in terms

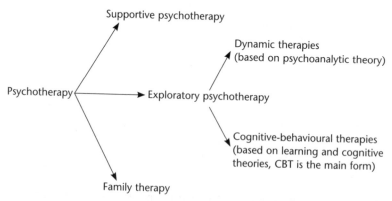

Figure 10.1 Cognitive behavioural therapy (CBT) in the context of psychotherapy as a whole. The three main forms of psychotherapy, supportive psychotherapy, exploratory psychotherapy (in the form of CBT), and family therapy can all have a role to play in the management of bipolar disorder. On balance, dynamic therapies based on psychoanalytic theory have not been proven effective in the management of bipolar disorder.

of his or her thoughts, emotions, and behaviour. This then leads to the identification of realistic, time-limited goals and of cognitive and behavioural strategies to achieve these goals. Negative or unhelpful thoughts are considered to be hypotheses that, through gentle questioning and guided discovery, can be examined, tested, and modified. Behavioural tasks include self-monitoring, activity scheduling, graded task assignments, and assertiveness training. In most cases, there is also an added focus on medication compliance and relapse prevention.

What are some of the thinking errors that occur in depression?

Some of the common thinking errors (or 'cognitive distortions') that occur in depression include:

- Arbitrary inference, which involves drawing a conclusion in the absence of evidence – an example would be, 'The whole world hates me.'
- Over-generalization, which involves drawing a conclusion on the basis of very limited evidence – an example would be, 'The shopkeeper gave me an angry look. The whole world hates me.'
- Magnification and minimization, which involve either over- or under-estimating the importance of an event – an example would be, 'The death of my cat means that I no longer have anything to look forward to.'
- Selective abstraction, which involves focusing on a single negative event or condition while ignoring other more positive ones – an example would be, 'I'm not in a relationship' – even though you have a supportive family and are good at making friends.
- Dichotomous thinking, which involves 'all-or-nothing' thinking – an example would be, 'If she doesn't come to see me today then she doesn't love me' – even though she's thinking about me all the time but has no transportation.
- Personalization, which involves relating independent events

to yourself – an example would be, 'The nurse left her job because she was fed up with me' – although she actually left for family reasons.

- Catastrophic thinking, which involves expecting disaster to strike at any minute – an example would be, 'If I go out to the post office this afternoon, I'm more than likely to get run over.'

What else can I do to fight off depression?

There are a number of simple things that you can do to fight off depression:

- Ask your doctor for help, and try to stick to any medication that he or she may prescribe.
- Break large tasks into small ones, set yourself realistic goals for completing them, and don't take on more than you can manage.
- Don't take any important decisions such as changing jobs or getting divorced while you are depressed. Thinking errors (see above) can lead you to make the wrong decision.
- Spend time with other people and talk to them about how you are feeling. You can also phone a helpline for practical advice and support (see Useful addresses, page 119).
- Let your family and friends help you. They may well be able to offer you the company, patience, affection, understanding, encouragement, and support that you need.
- Get out of the house, even if this is just to buy a pint of milk or take a walk in the park.
- Do more of the things that you usually enjoy doing: read a book, go to the shops or the cinema, visit friends – anything that takes your mind off your negative thoughts is likely to make you feel better.
- Take mild exercise.
- Get sufficient amounts of sleep. Even a single good night's sleep can make you feel much better.

- Use the techniques discussed in the previous section to reduce stress and anxiety.
- Fight your negative thoughts – perhaps the most important thing of all. Make a list of all the positive things about yourself (you may need to get help with this), keep it with you and read it to yourself several times a day. However bad you may be feeling, remember that you will not always be feeling this way. Have realistic expectations for yourself: improvements in mood are likely to be gradual rather than precipitous, and there are going to be both good days and bad days.

Agree whom to call if you feel overwhelmed by suicidal thoughts. This may be a relative or friend, a helpline, or your CMHT. Carry their telephone numbers with you.

Staying off alcohol and drugs

People with bipolar disorder who drink heavily or take illicit drugs are likely to suffer more frequent and more severe relapses in their illness. Those with depression may turn to alcohol or illicit drugs such as cannabis, amphetamines, or cocaine to obtain relief from their symptoms. Alcohol and drugs may temporarily blunt or mask symptoms, but in the long run they are likely to lead to more severe anxiety and depression, and to more frequent and severe relapses of bipolar illness. People can create a vicious circle in which the more they use alcohol and drugs to mask their symptoms, the worse their symptoms become, and the worse their symptoms become, the more they use alcohol and drugs. Alcohol and drugs may also delay them from getting help, including getting an all-important prescription for medication.

Apart from this, possible consequences of alcohol or drug use in bipolar disorder include:

- Increased psychotic symptoms
- Reduced response to medication

- Reduced compliance with medication
- Medical complications such as high blood pressure, heart attack, stroke, stomach ulcers, and liver disease
- Complications of intravenous drug use such as hepatitis, HIV infection, and venous thrombosis
- Family and marital difficulties
- Motoring offences
- Accidents
- Financial hardship
- Criminal activity and its consequences

Should you need it, simple advice and support is readily available from your CMHT. You may find it useful to ask a health-care professional to help you to devise a goal-oriented management plan tailored to your needs. Tasks in this management plan could in the first instance include, for example, keeping your appointments, keeping a diary of substance use, and taking your medication. Relatives can play an important role in supporting and monitoring progress and they should, if possible, be included in the management plan. They should try to adopt an open and non-judgmental approach in an attempt to bolster their loved one's self-esteem and make him or her feel in greater control of the problem.

Alcohol or drug use is often prompted by stressful situations, so learning techniques for managing stress and anxiety, such as deep breathing and progressive muscle relaxation, can be particularly helpful, as is learning and role-playing specific social skills, which can then be used in stressful and high-risk situations. Such social skills include saying 'no' to a drug dealer or going into a pub and ordering a non-alcoholic drink.

If you find yourself in a stressful situation and are about to give in to temptation, don't! Call a relative or carer, talk through the situation, and get the support and encouragement that you need to pull through. Some people with bipolar disorder also find support and encouragement in local support groups, or in more structured 12-step programmes such as Alcoholics Anonymous or Narcotics Anonymous. Ask your psychiatrist or key worker if such groups are suitable for you.

Alcoholics Anonymous

Founded in 1935 in Ohio, Alcoholics Anonymous is a spiritually oriented community of alcoholics whose aim is to stay sober and, through shared experience and understanding, to help other alcoholics to do the same, 'one day at a time', by avoiding that first drink. The essence of the programme involves a 'spiritual awakening' that is achieved by 'working the steps', usually with the guidance of a more experienced member or 'sponsor'. Members initially attend daily meetings in which they share their experiences of alcoholism and recovery and engage in prayer or meditation. A prayer that is usually recited at every meeting is the Serenity Prayer, the short version of which is:

> God grant me the serenity to accept the things I cannot change,
> Courage to change the things I can,
> And the wisdom to know the difference.

Taking care of your physical health

Bipolar disorder can encourage a number of unhealthy habits, and it also makes it difficult for you to start addressing these habits. Taking care of your physical health, however, not only increases life expectancy and quality of life, but also promotes recovery and fights off anxiety and depression. You create a 'virtuous circle' in which the better you feel, the better you are able to take care of your physical health, and the better you are able to take care of your physical health, the better you feel.

Compared with other groups of people, those with bipolar disorder are more likely to eat poorly, lack exercise, and smoke. For these reasons they are more likely to suffer from obesity, diabetes, cardiovascular problems such as high blood pressure, heart attack, and stroke, and respiratory problems such as chronic bronchitis and emphysema. Some of the possible side effects of medication (for example antipsychotic medication, lithium, or valproate) can directly or indirectly contribute to problems such as obesity and diabetes, making the care of your physical health all the more important.

Why do people with bipolar disorder often have poor physical health?

Some of the common reasons for poor physical health in people with bipolar disorder are:

- Poor diet
- Lack of exercise
- Smoking
- Alcohol and drug use
- Side effects of medication
- Social factors such as poor income and housing
- Poor monitoring of physical health

Physical health problems do not affect everyone with bipolar disorder, but it is important that you should have your physical health monitored so that any eventual problems can be detected early on. Your GP is normally able to carry out a physical check once every year. This usually involves weighing you, taking your pulse rate and blood pressure, and carrying out a blood or urine test. A physical check is a good opportunity to discuss your symptoms and medication, and to obtain advice on issues such as diet, exercise, and smoking. If you are on a mood stabilizer and require a blood test to monitor your physical health, this can usually be carried out in the same appointment.

Diet

There are two separate factors to consider about your diet:

- Whether you are eating the right amount to keep your weight in the desirable range for health
- Whether you are eating a healthy balanced diet

First, consult a height–weight chart (see Figure 10.2) to check whether you are the right weight for your height.

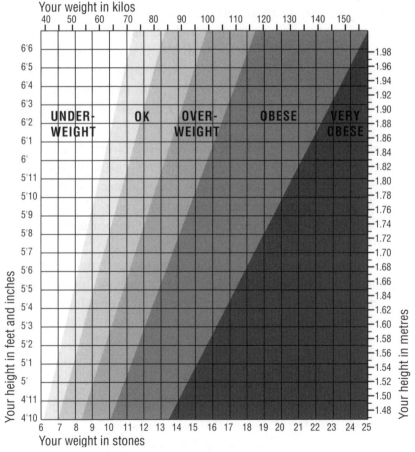

Figure 10.2 Height–weight chart.

If you are underweight for your height, this may be a cause for concern, and you should try to put on weight through eating sufficient quantities of a healthy, balanced diet. If this fails or if you are significantly underweight, you should consult your GP for further advice.

If you are overweight for your height, try to cut down on the amount that you are eating, especially on foods that are high in sugar or saturated and hydrogenated fats, and try to do more exercise. If you are fat or very fat for your height, you are at a high risk of physical health problems such as diabetes, high blood pressure, heart problems, and stroke. It is particularly important that you try to lose weight, but be realistic about what you can achieve: rather than go on to a 'crash diet' that is bound to end in failure, aim to lose small amounts of weight steadily over a longer period of time. Cut back on foods that are high in sugar or saturated and hydrogenated fats such as fried foods, meat products, hard cheese, cream, and butter. Eat three meals a day, but avoid snacking in between meals, especially on 'comfort' foods such as chocolate, cakes, biscuits, and crisps. If you do feel like snacking, have a piece of fruit such as an apple, pear, or banana. If you have had problems trying to lose weight in the past, consult your GP or a dietician for further advice.

If your weight is OK for your height, then you are eating about the right amount to keep your weight in the desirable range for health. This does not, however, mean that you are necessarily eating a healthy balanced diet.

What is a healthy balanced diet?

A healthy balanced diet:

- is based on starchy foods such as wholegrain bread, potatoes, pasta, and rice;
- contains a lot of fruit and vegetables (five portions a day);

- contains some protein-rich foods such as fish, poultry, meat, eggs, and pulses
- is low in fat, sugar, and salt

How do I maintain a healthy balanced diet?

Here are eight tips for eating well from eatwell, the UK Food Standards Agency consumer advice and information website <www.eatwell.gov.uk>:

1 Base your meals on starchy foods
2 Eats lots of fruits and vegetables
3 Eat more fish
4 Cut down on saturated fat and sugar
5 Try to eat less salt – no more than 6 grams a day
6 Get active and try to be a healthy weight
7 Drink plenty of water
8 Don't skip breakfast

If you are eating a healthy balanced diet, you are probably getting all the vitamins and minerals that your body needs, and you do not need to take any dietary supplements.

Exercise

Regular exercise is an important part of looking after both your physical and mental health. With regard to physical health, exercise helps you to lose weight and maintain your target weight once you have achieved it. It also decreases your blood pressure and increases your physical strength, endurance, and flexibility. Exercise usually improves the quality of your sleep, but it should not be taken just before bed time because its short-term alerting effects may prevent you from falling asleep.

With regard to mental health, exercise helps to decrease stress, improve thinking and motivation, boost self-esteem, and lift mood by causing the body to release increased amounts of chemical messengers called endorphins. Exercise also distracts you

Table 10.4   Some of the benefits of exercise in bipolar disorder

Weight loss

Improved physical strength, endurance, and flexibility

Decreased stress

Decreased blood pressure

Better sleep

Improved thinking

Improved motivation

Better mood

Better self-esteem

Distraction from psychotic symptoms

Removal from emotional conflict

Increased social interactions

from psychotic symptoms such as hallucinations and delusions, and it can also have a beneficial effect on these symptoms.

Exercise does not have to be difficult or intensive, and 30 minutes of moderate activity a day is all that is needed to improve your fitness. You could do some gardening, walk to the shops, cycle, exercise at a gym or swimming pool, or play a team sport such as basketball or football. In fact, there are so many possibilities to choose from that you are bound to find one that you enjoy doing. By getting you out of the house and 'out of yourself', exercise can remove you from emotional conflict, distract you from your symptoms, and increase the number and frequency of your social interactions. This in itself can have a beneficial effect on your mental health.

The particular benefits of exercise in people with bipolar disorder are summarized in Table 10.4.

Sleep

Loss of sleep or irregular sleep patterns can trigger a manic episode in people who have bipolar disorder or who are at risk of developing bipolar disorder. Even going to bed unusually late – for example, after having to meet an important deadline or after a big night out – can be sufficient to trigger a manic episode. For this reason, people with bipolar disorder who are students at university, work long hours, or work shifts are at particular risk of developing a manic episode. People with bipolar disorder may also develop a manic episode after travelling across several time zones and needing to readjust their internal clocks and sleep patterns. If a person's mood becomes even slightly abnormally elevated, he or she may be unable to sleep. As sleep is lost, his or her mood is likely to become even more abnormally elevated. As you can see, a vicious circle quickly takes hold. For

Table 10.5   Some of the more common causes of insomnia

Poor sleep habits

Psychiatric disorders
  Depressive disorder
  Bipolar disorder (mania and depression)
  Anxiety disorders
  Schizophrenia
  Post-traumatic stress disorder
  Chronic fatigue syndrome

Medical disorders
  Restless leg syndrome (causing thrashing about during sleep)
  Sleep apnoea (during sleep, snoring with pauses in breathing)
  Chronic pain
  Chronic obstructive pulmonary disease
  Chronic renal failure
  Neurological disorders such as Parkinson's disease and other movement
  disorders
  Headaches
  Fibromyalgia

Other
  Alcohol and drug misuse
  Side effects of medication such as antipsychotic or antidepressant
  medication
  Shift working
  Caring for young children

the person with bipolar disorder, it is all-important to recognize this vicious circle early and to cut it short.

Insomnia – difficulty in falling asleep or in staying asleep – affects about 30 per cent of the general population, but is even more common in those with bipolar disorder, in whom it can be a direct effect of the illness. Insomnia is usually a problem if it occurs on most nights and causes distress or daytime effects such as fatigue, poor concentration, poor memory, and irritability. These symptoms may not only delay your recovery but also predispose you to accidents, to anxiety and depression, and to medical disorders such as high blood pressure, infections, obesity, and diabetes. Insomnia can also be caused or aggravated by poor sleep habits, depression, anxiety, stress, physical problems such as pain or breathing problems, medication, and alcohol and drug use (see Table 10.5). Short-term insomnia specifically is often caused by a stressful life event, a poor sleeping environment, or an irregular routine.

If you are suffering from insomnia, there are a number of simple measures that you can take to resolve or at least lessen the problem:

- Have a strict routine involving regular and adequate sleeping times (most adults need about seven or eight hours of sleep every night). Allocate a time for sleeping, for example, 11.00 p.m. to 7.00 a.m., and do not use this time for any other activities. Avoid daytime naps, or make them short and regular. If you have a bad night, avoid 'sleeping in' because this makes it more difficult to fall asleep the following night.
- Have a relaxing bedtime routine that enables you to relax and 'wind down' before bedtime. This may involve doing breathing exercises or meditation (see page 84) or simply reading a book, listening to music, or watching TV.
- Many people find it helpful to have a hot drink: if this is the case for you, have a herbal or malted or chocolatey drink rather than stimulant drinks such as tea or coffee.

- Sleep in a familiar, dark, and quiet room that is adequately ventilated and neither too hot nor too cold. Try to use this room for sleeping only, so that you come to associate it with sleep.
- If you can't sleep, don't become anxious and try to force yourself to sleep. The more anxious you become, the less likely you are to fall asleep, and this is only likely to make you more anxious! Instead, get up and do something relaxing and enjoyable for about half an hour, and then try again.
- Take regular exercise during the daytime, but do not exercise in the evening or just before bedtime because the short-term alerting effects of exercise may make it more difficult for you to fall asleep.
- Try to reduce your overall levels of stress by implementing some of the lifestyle changes detailed on page 86.
- Eat an adequate evening meal containing a good balance of complex carbohydrates and protein. Eating too much can make it difficult to fall asleep; eating too little can disturb your sleep and decrease its quality.
- Avoid caffeine, alcohol, and tobacco, particularly in the evening. Also avoid stimulant drugs such as cocaine, amphetamines, and ecstasy. Alcohol may make you fall asleep more easily, but it decreases the quality of your sleep.

If insomnia persists despite these measures, seek advice from your GP or psychiatrist. In some cases, insomnia may have a clear and definite cause that needs to be addressed in itself – for example, a physical problem or a side effect of medication. Behavioural interventions such as sleep restriction therapy or cognitive behavioural therapy can be helpful in some cases and in the long term are preferable to sleeping tablets. Sleeping tablets can be effective in the short term but are best avoided in the longer term because of their side effects and their high potential for tolerance (meaning that you need progressively higher doses to achieve the same effect) and dependence.

Sleeping remedies that are available without a prescription often contain an antihistamine that can leave you feeling drowsy the following morning. If you decide to use such remedies, it is important that you do not drive or operate heavy machinery the next day. Herbal alternatives are usually based on the herb valerian, a hardy perennial flowering plant with heads of sweetly scented pink or white flowers. If you are thinking about using a herbal remedy, speak to your GP or psychiatrist first, particularly if you have a medical condition or allergy, are already on medication, or are pregnant or breast-feeding.

Smoking

People with bipolar disorder are much more likely to take up smoking than the average person. They are also more likely to smoke heavily, with dire consequences for their physical health, quality of life, and life expectancy. Indeed, cardiovascular and respiratory diseases that are both caused and aggravated by smoking are among some of the most common causes of death in bipolar sufferers. Smoking also results in a decrease in blood levels of antipsychotic medication, such that smokers require higher doses of antipsychotic medication than non-smokers to achieve the same therapeutic effect. And assuming that a pack of 20 cigarettes costs an average of £5.50, someone smoking 40 cigarettes a day spends $((£5.50) \times 2) \times 365 = £4,015$ on cigarettes each year. Although roll-up cigarettes are cheaper than filter cigarettes, they can also be more damaging to physical health.

Many people with bipolar disorder who smoke started smoking before their illness began, suggesting either that smoking predisposes to bipolar disorder or that the genetic or environmental factors that predispose to bipolar disorder also predispose to nicotine addiction. An alternative explanation for the high rates of smoking in people with bipolar disorder is that their illness makes them more likely to smoke, possibly because they feel that smoking enables them to relax or that it alleviates symptoms such as difficulty concentrating and hallucinations.

A commonly held perception is that people with bipolar disorder are unlikely to give up smoking and that it is unfair or even inhumane to try to deprive them of one of their principal pastimes and pleasures. The truth is that many people with bipolar disorder are themselves highly motivated to stop smoking and are in need of all the help that they can get to fight what is often a severe nicotine addiction. Help can take the form of smoking cessation groups, behavioural therapy, nicotine replacement (in the form of patches or lozenges, for example), and alternative therapies such as acupuncture and hypnosis. Success rates are highly variable from person to person, but it is important not to give up and to persist.

If you are motivated to stop smoking, mention this to your GP or psychiatrist. Further information and support is also available from <www.netdoctor.co.uk/smoking/index.shtml>.

How can I help myself to stop smoking?

Make a list of the pros and cons of smoking. See Table 10.6 for an example of such a list.

Keep your list with you and use it to motivate yourself to quit. Choose a date on which you want to quit and stick to it. Between now and that date keep a log of your smoking habits: record the times at which you 'light up', where you are, what you are doing, and how you are feeling. Use this log to gain a better understanding of your pattern of smoking. Once your chosen date arrives, make a clean break by throwing out all cigarettes and removing all ashtrays, lighters, and matches. You are likely to experience intense cravings and withdrawal symptoms such as irritability, difficulty concentrating, tiredness, headache, increased appetite, and insomnia. Nicotine replacement can help to relieve these cravings and withdrawal symptoms, so ask your GP or psychiatrist to prescribe them for you. Cravings rarely

Table 10.6   Pros and cons of smoking

Pros
Makes it easier to socialize with other smokers
Makes me feel more confident in social situations
Provides me with momentary gratification
Prevents cravings and withdrawal symptoms
Cons
Constant nagging from my partner
Bad breath putting my partner off
Constantly having to go outside, even in the cold and rain
The rancid smell in my house and on my clothes
The effects on my health: sore throat, cough, shortness of breath, high blood pressure, stomach ulcers
The effects on my appearance: looking 10 years older than I really am with yellow teeth, fingernails, and skin
Intense craving and withdrawal symptoms if I don't smoke
Always needing a fix, and being unable to simply relax and enjoy life
Feelings of inadequacy for not giving up
Feelings of fear and anxiety at what I am doing to myself and how it will all end
Feelings of guilt for the passive smoking endured by those around me
The cost of it all, especially the fact that I can never afford a holiday

last for more than a couple of minutes at a time, so diversion techniques such as chewing gum, brushing your teeth, or doing a crossword puzzle may take your mind off them until they pass. If these diversion techniques fail, call a friend or relative who knows what you are going through and has agreed to offer you help and support. Alternatively, read your list of pros and cons and use it to keep yourself motivated. Cravings are often triggered by certain places, activities, and emotions that you have learned to associate with smoking. Use the log of your smoking habits to identify these places, activities, and emotions, and try to think of alternative coping strategies to smoking.

Remember that cravings and withdrawal symptoms do not last for ever, and that in a matter of only days quitting will have become a much easier task! Don't be too harsh on yourself if you give in to temptation: put it behind you and keep on trying your best.

Coping with stigma

One of the most difficult challenges in recovering from bipolar disorder is coping with the reactions of other people. Mental illness in general and psychotic illnesses in particular are heavily stigmatized by the general public. This is in large part due to ignorance and the fear that is born out of it, a fear that is sadly reinforced by the misrepresentation of people with psychotic illnesses in the media. People with bipolar disorder do not have split personalities, and as a group they are neither unpredictable nor dangerous. They are not lazy or 'moral failures', and getting better is not simply a matter of them 'pulling themselves together'. Mental illnesses, like all medical conditions, have a biological basis and are not simply 'in the mind'.

It has been suggested that the genes that predispose to bipolar disorder also confer an important adaptive advantage to mankind, namely, the ability for language and creativity. Some highly creative people have or have had bipolar disorder, including most probably Lord Byron, Edgar Allen Poe, Vincent van Gogh, Virginia Woolf, Ernest Hemingway, Kurt Cobain, and Stephen Fry. Similarly, many highly creative people have had close relatives affected by bipolar disorder and other mental illnesses.

Stigma can create a vicious circle of alienation and discrimination that hinders progress to recovery by promoting social isolation, stress, depression, alcohol and drug misuse, unemployment, homelessness, and institutionalization. Sadly, many people with bipolar disorder report that the stigma attached to mental illness is just as distressing as its actual symptoms. In some cases people fear stigma to such an extent that they find it difficult to accept that they are ill, and as a result do not seek out or accept the help that they need. For these reasons it is particularly important that carers analyse their attitudes and behaviours, and ensure that they are not involuntarily contributing to the stigma felt by the person that they are caring for. Attitudes and behaviours that contribute to stigma are often subtle, and may, for example, involve talking to people with bipolar disorder as if they are children or hard of hearing, talking about them as if they are not in the room, and failing to grant them sufficient independence and responsibility. A simple rule of thumb for carers is to behave towards the person with bipolar disorder as they would towards any other person: naturally, simply, and with due respect and courtesy. Carers should try to be a 'refuge' or 'comfort zone' for the person that they are caring for, offering him or her practical and emotional support, but also the space and time to be quiet and alone. Deep questioning, argument and the venting of intense negative emotions may overwhelm the person with bipolar disorder and definitely need to be avoided.

Many people with bipolar disorder feel unable to talk about their illness for fear of the pain and shame of being stigmatized. Being open about your illness may be a risk, but it also enables you to talk about your feelings and gain the support that you need. Learn as much as you can about your illness, so that you yourself can correct any false beliefs that people may hold about it. Try to educate friends and relatives about bipolar disorder and the issues surrounding it. If people use derogatory terms such as 'maniac' or 'psycho', remind them that their behaviour is unacceptable. If you feel that you are being unfairly treated as a customer or service user, make a complaint. You can even take a public stance against discrimination – for example, by speaking at events or writing about your experiences on a blog or in a local newspaper or magazine. Joining a local support group enables you to meet other people with bipolar disorder and, at least temporarily, escape stigma. You can also use support groups to share your experiences and learn from and support one another.

Preventing relapses

Relapses can have devastating consequences for the person with bipolar disorder and for his or her relatives and friends. After each relapse it may become increasingly difficult to regain control over the symptoms, and this affects not only long-term outcome but also quality of life. For these reasons, it is particularly important to prevent relapses as best as possible.

There is strong scientific evidence that long-term treatment with medication substantially reduces rates of relapse and re-hospitalization in bipolar disorder. If you are reluctant to take your medication because the schedule is too complicated or because you are suffering from side effects that you find unacceptable, speak to your psychiatrist about it. Your psychiatrist may be able to simplify the schedule, decrease the dose, or change you to another medication that suits you better. **Do not simply stop taking your medication.** Taking your medication at the dose prescribed by your psychiatrist is often the single most important thing you can do to prevent a relapse. People with bipolar disorder and their carers should learn to recognize the early signs and symptoms of a relapse. These signs and symptoms may differ from person to person, but common ones include:

- Suffering changes in mood
- Losing your sense of humour
- Becoming tense, irritable or agitated
- Finding it difficult to concentrate
- Retreating from social situations and neglecting outside activities and social relationships
- Saying or doing irrational or inappropriate things
- Developing strange or unbelievable ideas

- Neglecting your personal care
- Neglecting to take your medication
- Dressing in unusual clothes or in unusual combinations of clothes
- Sleeping excessively or hardly at all
- Eating excessively or hardly at all
- Becoming increasingly suspicious or hostile
- Becoming especially sensitive to noise or light
- Hearing voices or seeing things that other people cannot hear or see.

If any of these signs and symptoms should arise, contact your local mental health-care team as soon as possible for support and advice as this may help in averting a full-scale relapse. It is a good idea to have an action plan in place before problems arise and to have discussed this plan with your local mental health-care team. You can also keep a diary to help you to identify the signs and symptoms of a relapse, should one arise. Remember that a relapse may impair your thinking and prevent you from recognizing those signs and symptoms. You may therefore need to rely on family and friends, and to trust in their judgement.

Table 10.7 Some of the most important factors that may cause or contribute to a relapse of bipolar disorder

Poor understanding of bipolar disorder in general, and symptoms of relapse in particular

Non-compliance with medication or decreased dose of medication (see page 107)

Drugs and alcohol (see page 91)

Lack of sleep or irregular pattern of sleep (see page 98)

Stress (see page 81)

Lack of social relationships and support

Stigma (see page 105)

Poor physical health (see page 93)

Try to identify any factors that may have caused or contributed to your difficulties, as addressing these factors may help you to avert a full-scale relapse. Some of the most important of these factors are listed in Table 10.7 and discussed more fully in other sections of this book. Minimizing them can help you to prevent relapses and significantly improve your chances of a durable recovery.

Driving and bipolar disorder

You should stop driving during a first episode or relapse of your illness, because driving can seriously endanger lives. In the UK, you must notify the Driver and Vehicle Licensing Agency (DVLA). Failure to do so makes it illegal for you to drive and invalidates your insurance. The DVLA then sends you a medical questionnaire to fill in, and a form asking for your permission to contact your psychiatrist. Your driving licence can generally be reinstated if your psychiatrist can confirm that:

- Your illness has been successfully treated with medication for a period of at least three months (six months in rapid cycling)
- You are conscientious about taking your medication
- The side effects of your medication are not likely to impair your driving
- You are not misusing drugs

Further information on bipolar disorder and driving can be obtained from the DVLA website at <www.DVLA.gov.uk>. Note that the rules for professional driving are different from those described above.

11

Caring for carers

According to Carers UK, each year in the UK over two million people take up a caring role, so you are certainly not alone. A good carer can be the most valuable source of structure and support for a person with bipolar disorder, and his or her greatest hope for a permanent recovery. Though you may feel that caring for a loved one is more a duty than a job, it is important that you identify yourself as a carer so as to obtain the help and support that all people in a caring role need.

Try to learn as much as you can about bipolar disorder and to have a good idea of how it might affect the person that you are caring for. For example, the person that you are caring for may sometimes not be spontaneous in his or her responses to your questions. It may feel as if he or she is ignoring you, but it is in fact because he or she is being distracted by voices. Understanding the illness builds up your confidence as a carer and gives you a clearer sense of what you might be able to achieve. Remember that there is only so much you alone can do to help the person you are caring for: being realistic about how much you can achieve enables you to prevent conflict, manage stress, and avoid burn-out. Speak to your local mental health-care team for further information about bipolar disorder and for specific advice about caring for your relative. Information and advice is also available from voluntary organizations such as the ones listed at the back of this book (see Useful addresses, page 119).

Caring for a person with bipolar disorder is likely to require a lot of patience: during a relapse, people with bipolar disorder may have good days and bad days and tend to make progress in only small steps. A relapse is likely to sap your morale, but it is important that you be prepared for this. It is a good idea to have an action plan in place before problems arise, and to have discussed it with your local mental health-care team. If problems arise, contact the mental health-care team sooner rather than later, because doing so may prevent any problems from getting worse. Remember that your caring role has made you an important source of information and expertise: learn to rely on your previous experiences and to trust in your judgement. At the same time, try to involve the person you are caring for in making decisions about his or her care.

Sometimes a person with bipolar disorder may fail to recognize that he or she is ill, and so refuse to engage with the mental health-care team. In particular, he or she may insist that delusions and hallucinations are real or may be too paranoid to trust in carers. If the person is refusing to engage with the mental health-care team, carers can try breaking the prospect of treatment into smaller, more manageable steps, starting with an initial appointment. If possible, give the person a degree of choice in booking the appointment, and propose that you or someone else goes along to the appointment.

As progress tends to be made in only small steps, it is easy for carers to lose sight of the fact that progress is actually being made. Try to feel positive about the person that you are caring for and gently encourage and facilitate his or her progress. One of the most important things you can do as a carer is to ensure that the person you are caring for takes his or her medication as prescribed. Be on the lookout for any potential side effects, and do not hesitate to report them to your local mental health-care team. Try to establish and maintain a simple daily structure and routine involving regular meal times and sleeping times for the person you are caring for. Gently encourage him or her to attend appointments with members of the mental health-care team and other services.

Avoid nagging, criticizing, telling off, shouting, and arguing. Do not lose sight of the fact that stress is an important predictor of relapse in bipolar disorder, and ensure that you are giving the person you are caring for sufficient time and space to get better. This can be difficult to achieve, because it is often a carer's instinct to try to do as much as possible for the person being cared for, and many carers have unrealistic expectations about the progress that their loved one with bipolar disorder ought to be making. If you feel that this is an issue for you and the person that you are caring for, speak to your local mental health-care team about it. Families with these kinds of issue can be offered educational sessions, stress management, or family therapy: these can all help to reduce stress and can be important and integral parts of the care plan.

Finally, do not neglect other family members. Brothers and sisters of people with bipolar disorder, particularly if they are young, may feel that they are not getting their fair share of your attention and may become jealous and resentful.

Look after your physical and mental health

Carers need to care for themselves if they are to care most effectively for a significant other. Many carers come under severe stress and as a result suffer from serious health problems such as heart disease or mental illness. It is important that you recognize this and take it seriously if you are not to become ill and unable to fulfil your carer role. Use some of the techniques for stress management listed on page 86 to reduce your levels of stress, and arrange for an annual health check-up to be carried out by your GP. Make sure that you look after yourself, that you plan and pursue activities that you enjoy, and that you take a break or holiday from caring if you feel that you need one.

Get the emotional support that you need

Remember that you are not alone as a carer: share your opinions and experiences with the mental health-care team looking after the person you are caring for, and ask them for help and advice. Conversely, your perspective on the person that you are caring for is invaluable to the team, so try to attend and participate in the regularly held CPA meetings. Identify someone that you can talk to on a more personal level – perhaps a close relative or friend – about your experiences as a carer. Many family members and friends may find it difficult to discuss your caring role, and tend to underestimate the effort that you are making as a carer. The onus is on you to broach the subject and enlist their help and support. Joining a local carers' support group enables you to feel that you are not alone in your carer role, and such a support group can provide a valuable opportunity to learn from the experiences of other carers.

Joining a carers' support group can also help you to understand any negative emotions that you may be harbouring, such as guilt, shame, and anger, and to prevent these emotions from affecting the person that you are caring for.

Avoid blaming yourself or others

Parents sometimes think that bipolar disorder is caused by bad parenting, and fear that they may be to blame for their son or daughter's illness. Their feelings of guilt can come to dominate family life, and simply add to the heavy burden already carried by their son or daughter. In the 1940s some psychoanalysts believed that certain mental illnesses such as schizophrenia and autism resulted from having a so-called 'refrigerator mother', an emotionally absent and therefore inadequate mother. This theory and other similar theories have never found scientific backing, and have long since been discredited and discarded. In fact, scientific research is quite clear about the fact that bipolar disorder is a biological illness of the brain.

Parents also sometimes look around for someone else to blame for their son or daughter's illness, such as the GP, the psychiatrist, or even their son or daughter. That they should do so is natural and understandable since it helps them to make sense of the illness of a loved one. Nevertheless, it is important that they should remember that the real 'culprit' is ultimately a biological illness of the brain. They should avoid playing the 'blame game' and instead focus their energies on the challenging journey to recovery.

Like guilt and blame, frustration and anger can be a normal reaction to the illness of a loved one. Parents also often have thoughts such as, 'Why did this happen to our family?' or even, 'Why should I even bother? It's too much hard work and, ultimately, it's all going to be for nothing.' Sometimes parents may direct their anger and frustration at their son or daughter, even though they realize that he or she is not to blame for the illness. Unchecked anger adds to your stress and to that of your son or daughter, and thereby prevents your family from moving ahead. Although you cannot change the reality of the illness, you can change your reaction to it. Try diffusing your anger by being honest and open about the feelings that underlie it: talk to relatives, friends, mental health-care professionals, and other families affected by bipolar disorder. Or else try channelling your anger so that it becomes a force for the good – for example, by motivating you to seek out help for your family.

Get the practical support that you need

You can obtain an assessment of your needs as a carer by asking your GP to refer you to local Social Services or by referring yourself directly to them. A carer's needs assessment is often helpful in ensuring that your practical needs as a carer are met. You can find out about the carer support services available in your area through Social Services, through a local carers' organization, or through Carers UK and their dedicated phone line, CarersLine (see Useful addresses, page 119). Such services may include, among other things, help at home, the provision of aids and equipment, break services, and day care. Many carers are reluctant to claim social benefits, either because they have never done so before or because they are put off by the complicated rules and difficult forms.

As a carer you play an important role in society, and the benefits that you are entitled to exist to recognize and support that role. Some of these benefits are detailed on page 117, and you can obtain help in claiming them from your local mental health-care team, local Social Services, or voluntary organizations such as Carers UK.

Your life outside your caring role

Being a carer is highly stressful and it can become all-encompassing. It is very important that you think about yourself and your future, because a time may come when you are no longer required to be a carer. As the condition of the person you are caring for improves, he or she may become more independent and in some cases may move out to a place of his or her own. When this happens carers often find themselves lacking in purpose and direction, and unable to adjust to their changed circumstances. For this and other reasons it is vital that you continue to plan and pursue activities that you enjoy, and that you keep up your life outside your caring role. Many carers are able to be employed in a part-time job, and this can be both a salutatory distraction from the stress of caring and an invaluable source of additional income. Similarly, some carers are able to further their skills, for example by enrolling on an evening course or by studying part-time for a degree.

Siblings

As parents focus their attention on their ill son or daughter, they run the risk of becoming less available to their other children. These children are also in need of parental attention, since they are likely to have been profoundly affected by the illness of their brother or sister. They may be anxious for their family and fearful of developing the illness themselves. Bipolar disorder often strikes in the prime of life, at a time when young people are launching into life – starting college or university, getting a first job, or enjoying an expanding range of activities and relationships. For this reason, siblings may find it particularly difficult to enjoy their successes while witnessing their ill brother or sister slipping further and further behind. At the same time, they may feel pressured to achieve more so as to 'compensate' for their brother or sister's illness and not to add to the concerns of their afflicted parents.

Siblings should not blame themselves or anybody else for their brother or sister's illness or let it prevent them from enjoying their life outside of the family. By nurturing outside friendships, they may be able to obtain support and talk through difficult feelings such as anger, anxiety, and guilt. Parents need to make a special effort to remember the needs of siblings, and to ensure as far as possible that they are included in family discussions surrounding the illness. Siblings should educate themselves as much as possible about bipolar disorder, and also consider joining a carers' support group. Older siblings may be able to play an active role in caring and in due course become an invaluable source of support and respite to their parents. If siblings feel that they are not getting the parental attention that they need, they should not feel afraid to ask for it.

Social benefits

Every year in the UK millions of pounds of benefits are left un-claimed, often by people with a mental illness and their carers. Some of the benefits available to people with a mental illness and their carers are detailed here. For further information on these benefits, see the Department for Work and Pensions website, <www.dwp.gov.uk/lifeevent/benefits>, contact your local Citizens Advice Bureau, or get in touch with local Social Services.

Housing benefit and council tax benefit

Housing benefit and council tax benefit are means-tested, tax-free payments made to people who need help paying their rent and their council tax, respectively. Both benefits are administered by the local authority in whose area the property is situated. These benefits do not cover mortgage interest payments.

Income support

Income support is a means-tested payment made to people who are between the ages of 16 and 59 who work fewer than 16 hours a week and who have a reason for not actively seeking work (on grounds of disability, caring for children, or caring for relatives). Claimants of income support are also entitled to other benefits such as housing benefit and council tax benefit (see above).

Social fund

Social fund payments are payments, grants, or loans made in addition to certain benefits for important intermittent expenses that cannot be met by normal income.

Incapacity benefit

Incapacity benefit is paid to people who cannot work because of illness or disability and who cannot get statutory sick pay from their employer. It is related to national insurance contributions and requires regular medical certificates. It is not means-tested.

Disabled person's tax credit

The disabled person's tax credit is for people over the age of 16 who work an average of 16 hours a week or more and who have an illness or disability that restricts the amount that they can earn.

Disability living allowance

Disability living allowance is paid to people under the age of 65 who are in need of personal care or help with getting around, or both. It is not means-tested.

Attendance allowance

Attendance allowance is paid to people aged 65 or more who need help with personal care because of an illness or disability. It is not means-tested.

NHS costs

Depending on your circumstances you may qualify for free NHS prescriptions and hospital medicines, free NHS dental treatment, and free NHS eyesight tests. Other NHS costs may be met too.

Carer's allowance

Carer's allowance is a means-tested, taxable weekly benefit payment made to people who look after someone who is receiving Attendance Allowance or Disability Living Allowance at the middle or high rate of care. Among other stipulations, the carer must be over 16 years of age and spend 35 hours a week or more in his or her caring role. The carer does not have to be related to or living with the person he or she is caring for.

Useful addresses

MDF The BiPolar Organisation
Castle Works
21 St George's Road
London SE1 6ES
Tel.: 08456 340 540
Website: www.mdf.org.uk

MDF the BiPolar Organisation works to enable people affected by bipolar disorder (formerly known as manic depression) to take control of their lives by: expanding and developing information services about the condition; supporting and developing self-help opportunities, including self-help groups; decreasing discrimination against people with bipolar disorder, and promoting their social inclusion and rights; and influencing the improvement of treatments and services that aid recovery.

SANE
First Floor, Cityside House
40 Adler Street
London E1 1EE
Tel.: 020 7375 1002 (administration)
SANEline: 0845 767 8000 (6 p.m. to 11 p.m. every day including Sundays and public holidays, charged at local rates throughout the UK; calls can be anonymous and their contents are confidential)
Website: www.sane.org.uk

The work of SANE includes: campaigning for better services and treatments for people with serious mental illness and undertaking research into the causes of it; and providing information, crisis care and emotional support to those with mental-health problems and their families and carers through SANEline.

Mind (National Association for Mental Health)
15–19 Broadway
London E15 4BQ
MindinfoLine: 0845 766 0163 (9 a.m. to 5 p.m., Monday to Friday, charged at local rates throughout the UK)
Website: www.mind.org.uk

Mind's work includes: advancing the views, needs and ambitions of people with mental-health problems, challenging discrimination against them and campaigning for their rights; and raising public awareness of mental-health issues.

Rethink (formerly the National Schizophrenia Fellowship)
28 Castle Street
Kingston-upon-Thames KT1 1SS
Tel.: 0845 456 0455 (general enquiries)
National Advice Service: 020 8974 6814 (10 a.m. to 3 p.m., Monday,
Wednesday, Friday; 10 a.m. to 1 p.m., Tuesday, Thursday)
Website: www.rethink.org

Rethink offers over 350 services and more than 130 support groups
nationally. The range of services includes advocacy, carer support,
community support, employment and training, helplines, housing,
nursing and residential care, and services dedicated to black and minority
ethnic communities. The organization also produces a quarterly magazine,
Your Voice, and a range of other publications, many available through the
Mental Health Shop, an online resource that Rethink helped to set up in
2006 for booklets, leaflets, videos, DVDs etc. (<wwwmentalhealthshop.
org.>).

Making Space
Lyne House
46 Allen Street
Warrington
Cheshire WA2 7JB
Tel.: 01925 571680
Website: www.makingspace.co.uk

Making Space exists to improve the long-term welfare of people with
mental-health difficulties and those who care for them. The current area
of operation includes Cheshire, Cumbria, Greater Manchester, Lancashire,
Merseyside, Staffordshire and Yorkshire. In addition to family and carer
support, services offered include befriending schemes, day centres,
education and training schemes, residential care homes, supported
housing schemes, and short breaks and holidays.

Depression Alliance
212 Spitfire Studios
63–71 Collier Street
London N1 9BE
Tel.: 0845 123 23 20
Website: www.depressionalliance.org

Depression Alliance, the leading UK charity for people with depression,
provides publications, supporter services, local self-help groups and a
pen-friend scheme; researches into depression and works towards raising
public awareness of the condition; and campaigns for changes to mental-
health policy and practices.

Carers UK
20 Great Dover Street
London SE1 4LX
Tel.: 020 7378 4999
CarersLine: 0808 808 7777 (free, 10 a.m. to 12 p.m., Wednesdays and Thursdays)
Website: www.carersuk.org

Carers give so much to society yet, as a consequence, they can experience ill health, poverty and discrimination; and this organization works to end this injustice in the following ways: it mobilizes carers and supporters; campaigns for change; transforms understanding of caring; carries out research; and provides information and advice to carers through the CarersLine.

Samaritans
Chris
PO Box 9090
Stirling FK8 2SA
Helpline: 08457 90 90 90 (charged at local rates throughout the UK; 24 hours a day, every day of the year).
Website: www.samaritans.org.uk

In Samaritans' own words: 'We are always here to listen. Call us. It doesn't matter who you are – if you are in crisis, despairing or suicidal, contact us. It can make all the difference to talk about how you are feeling. You can speak in total confidence with one of our volunteers about anything that is troubling you. We will not judge you; we will not tell you what to do; but we will try to help you think things through. With Samaritans, you get the time and the space to find a way through. We will be there for you, to listen with an open mind for as long as you need.' Writing to the address above is an alternative for those who find telephones daunting.

Drinkline
Freephone 0800 917 8282

This National Alcohol Helpline is a confidential service that offers information and support to callers, and their relatives and friends.

Alcoholics Anonymous
PO Box 1
10 Toft Green
York YO1 7ND
Helpline: 0845 769 7555 (24 hours)
Website: www.alcoholics-anonymous.org.uk

Alcoholics Anonymous is a spiritually oriented community of alcoholics whose aim is to stay sober and, through shared experience and understanding, to help other alcoholics to do the same, 'one day at a time', by avoiding that first drink. The essence of the programme involves a 'spiritual awakening' that is achieved by 'working the steps', usually with the guidance of a more experienced member of 'sponsor'. Members initially attend daily meetings in which they share their experiences of alcoholism and recovery and engage in prayer and meditation.

Al-Anon
61 Great Dover Street
London SE1 4YF
Tel.: 020 7403 0888 (helpline, 10 a.m. to 10 p.m., 365 days a year)
Website: www.al-anonuk.org.uk

Offers understanding and support for families and friends of problem drinkers. At Al-Anon group meetings members receive comfort and understanding and learn to cope with their problems through the exchange of experience, strength and hope. Members learn that there are things that they can do to help themselves and, indirectly, to help the problem drinker.

QUIT
211 Old Street
London EC1V 9NR
Quitline: 0800 00 22 00
Website: www.quit.org.uk
Email: stopsmoking@quit.org.uk

QUIT's mission statement says that the organization's aim is to provide practical help, advice and support to all smokers who want to stop. Services include the Quitline for free help and advice, and counselling via email.

Cocaine Anonymous UK (CAUK)
PO Box 46920
London E2 9WF
Helpline: 0800 612 0225 (10 a.m. to 10 p.m., 365 days a year)
Website: www.cauk.org.uk

CAUK is a fellowship of men and women who share their experience, strength and hope with one another so that they may solve their common problem and help others to recover from their addiction. The only requirement for membership is a desire to stop using cocaine and all other mind-altering substances.

Sleep Council
High Corn Mill
Chapel Hill
Skipton
N. Yorkshire BD23 1NL
Tel.: 0845 058 4595 (admin)
Freephone leaflet line: 0800 018 7923
Website: www.sleepcouncil.com

The Sleep Council provides useful advice about sleep and about choosing a bed.

CRISIS
66 Commercial Street
London E1 6LT
Helpline: 0844 251 0111
Website: www.crisis.org.uk

CRISIS provides help and support to homeless people and people in danger of becoming homeless, so that they can rebuild their lives and not remain trapped in the cycle of homelessness.

Royal College of Psychiatrists
17 Belgrave Square
London SW1X 8PG
Tel.: 020 7235 2351
Website: www.rcpsych.ac.uk/mentalhealthinformation.aspx

This is the professional and educational organization for psychiatrists in the UK and Ireland. It produces a range of high-quality publications for general information, including various leaflets on bipolar disorder and treatments such as cognitive behavioural therapy and depot medication.

Mental Health Act
To help people find their way around this, Mr Nigel Turner has set up a succinct internet guide, *Hyper*GUIDE. It is free to users.
Website: www.hyperguide.co.uk/mha

Index